Cancer Care
and Cost
DRGs and Beyond

Cancer Care

and Cost DRGs and Beyond

Richard M. Scheffler and Neil C. Andrews
Editors

Kathryn A. Phillips
Associate Editor

Health Administration Press Perspectives
Ann Arbor, Michigan   1989

94 93 92 91 90   5 4 3 2 1

Library of Congress Cataloging-in-Publication Data

Cancer care and cost : DRGs and beyond / Richard M. Scheffler
    and Neil C. Andrews, editors ; Kathryn A. Phillips, associate
    editor.
    p.   cm.
    Based on a conference in 1987, sponsored by the American
Cancer Society, California Division.
    Includes bibliographical references.
    ISBN 0-910701-45-8 (soft)
    1. Cancer—Treatment—Economic aspects—United States—
Congresses.   2. Cancer—Patients—Medical care—United
States—Costs—Congresses.   3. Aged—Medical care—United
States—Costs—Congresses.   4. Diagnosis related groups—
United States—Congresses.   I. Scheffler, Richard M.
II. Andrews, Neil C.   III. Phillips, Kathryn A.   IV. American
Cancer Society. California Division.
    [DNLM: 1. Costs and Cost Analysis—congresses.
2. Diagnostic Related Groups—congresses.   3. Insurance,
Health—Economics—United States—congresses.   4. Medical
Oncology—economics—congresses.   5. Neoplasms—prevention
& control—congresses.   QZ 200 C2151207 1987]
RC270.8.C343   1989   338.4'7362196994'00973—dc20
DNLM/DLC for Library of Congress   89 – 19803 CIP

Health Administration Press
A Division of the Foundation of the
   American College of Healthcare Executives
1021 East Huron Street
Ann Arbor, Michigan 48104 – 9990
(313)764 – 1380

This book is for my father Benjamin, who, as a cancer patient, understands the issues raised from a unique perspective.

Richard M. Scheffler

To the staff and volunteers of the California Division of the American Cancer Society and to Carla.

Neil C. Andrews

To my professors and mentors, both at school and in life.

Kathryn A. Phillips

Table of Contents

List of Figures

List of Tables

Foreword

Cancer is a serious health problem in the United States. The American Cancer Society estimates that 1,540,000 new cases of cancer will occur in 1988. Among them, 555,000 will be nonmelanomatous skin cancers and in situ carcinomas of the uterus, cervix, and breast. A 100 percent cure rate can be expected with appropriate treatment of these three types of cancer. A 50 percent cure rate will be achieved in the 985,000 new cases of other types of cancer (American Cancer Society 1988).

In its 1988 annual review of cancer statistics, the National Cancer Institute reports upon the trends in cancer incidence, mortality, and survival between 1950 and 1985. Age-adjusted cancer incidence rates have risen 36.5 percent, from 270.6 cases per 100,000 in 1950 to 369.4 per 100,000 in 1985. Mortality rates have risen from 157.2 per 100,000 in 1950 to 167.8 per 100,000 in 1985, a 6.7 percent increase. However, five-year survival rates have improved 28.1 percent, from 39.1 percent to 50.1 percent during this period (National Cancer Institute 1988).

By the year 2010, 25 percent of Americans will be 55 years of age or older (American Cancer Society 1987). This age group has the highest overall incidence and mortality rate from cancer. It is estimated that the average time from exposure to a carcinogen to the development of cancer is 15 to 20 years (Greenwald and Sondik 1986). Unless some unforeseeable major research advance occurs in cancer prevention, the number of individuals with cancer will continue to rise. Cancer may become the leading cause of death and certainly will continue to be a major health problem for the United States in the next century.

The costs of medical care represent a staggering burden to the American people, consuming more than 11 percent of our gross national product. Medical care costs more than $1 billion per day (Health Care Financing Administration 1987). Cancer is among the most costly of all illnesses, accounting for 5 percent of our health expenditures. When the indirect costs of morbidity and mortality are added to the expenditures for direct health care, the cost of cancer to our society is nearly $70,000 for each new case (Ad Hoc Group for Medical Research Funding 1988).

With the development of new and better treatments, cancer survival has steadily improved. More than 5,000,000 Americans who have had cancer are alive today. Three million of them have lived more than five years after diagnosis and are considered cured (American Cancer Society 1988). This improved survival rate has resulted from better detection, evaluation, treatment, and rehabilitation. The goal, of course, is to provide all of these services appropriately and return the cancer patient to a normal, productive role in society. Refinement of cancer management has occurred at an ever-increasing cost to the patient and society. Unfortunately, society is facing a major confrontation between the rising costs for cancer care and our ability to pay for them. The socioeconomic, medical, and ethical issues involved in all health care delivery must be carefully reviewed before we can decide how to allocate our national resources.

With considerable foresight, the California Division of the American Cancer Society began planning several years ago for a conference to address these important issues. The planners agreed to bring together leaders with expertise in various aspects of health care delivery to review and discuss key issues regarding cancer care and cost. The conference, "Cancer Care and Cost: DRGs and Beyond," was held on May 29–30, 1987 in Coronado, California. The papers and discussion presented at that conference form the nucleus of this book.

The chapters in Part I discuss the economic burden of cancer care on our society today and the impact that reimbursement by diagnosis-related groups (DRGs) has had on this care. They express concern about the broader question of how we, as a society, should allocate our resources to achieve the maximum benefit for all of our citizens. Our present patterns of reimbursement for medical care do not support the overall objectives in cancer control. The payment mechanism was designed to reimburse hospitals, physicians, and others for treatment of disease rather than for primary or secondary prevention of disease, yet support for prevention could lead to substantial gains against cancer.

Part II focuses on the costs of cancer care for patients of different ages and different stages of cancer. The initial cost of cancer care is markedly less than the costs of terminal care. Nearly 6 percent of all annual expenditures of Medicare go to cancer patients in their last year of life. This expenditure is markedly influenced by such factors as geographic location and hospice use.

Parts III and IV explore the dilemma between cost of health care and quality of care. The authors demonstrate that these two concepts are not necessarily synonymous. Most authorities agree that high-quality care increases expenses. When health care providers are confronted with a choice between control of costs and maintenance of quality of care, they face an enormous ethical dilemma. The outcome of this conflict between quality and cost of care can be decided only when all sectors of society have provided input into the final decision.

In response to the problem of providing increasing reimbursement for the spiraling costs of health care, government representatives, health care providers, and insurance representatives have outlined a variety of issues we must face in the future. The three chapters in Part V address these issues. Costs may be lowered by increased use of outpatient care. "Prospective management" of cases is likely to optimize quality and contain costs of care. A strong recommendation has been made for the support of health services research, since more knowledge is needed before appropriate decisions can be made about future financing of health care delivery.

The two chapters in Part VI address moral and ethical issues such as access to health care, the inability of a large segment of society to gain access to appropriate medical care, and the complex dilemma of allocating limited resources to the delivery of quality health care. One interesting discussion centers on the use of volunteerism to expand the availability of health care resources. Acceptance of this concept would certainly support the role of organizations such as the American Cancer Society in the overall effort toward cancer control.

The time has clearly passed when we can give to everyone all the modern, technologically advanced medical care available. As we face the future, all Americans must take responsibility in determining who will receive our limited health care benefits. To do this, we surely want to achieve the most benefit per dollar spent. This book contains a clear assessment of the current status of cancer care costs and predictions for changes in the future. Everyone involved in the field of cancer care will benefit by reading it.

Harmon J. Eyre, M.D.
Immediate Past President
American Cancer Society

REFERENCES

Ad Hoc Group for Medical Research Funding. (1988). *Diseases and Disorders: The Human and Economic Cost.* Bethesda, MD: Ad Hoc Group for Medical Research Funding.

American Cancer Society. (1987). "Report of the Ad Hoc Committee on Strategic Planning." New York: American Cancer Society.

_____. (1988). *Cancer Facts and Figures – 1988.* New York: American Cancer Society.

Greenwald, P., and Sondik, E., eds. (1986). *Cancer Control Objectives for the Nation: 1985 – 2000.* PHS Publication 86 – 2880. National Cancer Institute. Bethesda, MD: National Institutes of Health.

Health Care Financing Administration. (1987). "National Health Expenditures, 1986 – 2000," *Health Care Financing Review* 8(4):1 – 36.

National Cancer Institute. (1988). *1988 Annual Cancer Statistics Review Including Cancer Trends: 1950 – 1985.* Bethesda, MD: National Institutes of Health.

Preface

The health services researcher, who works in a field that is marked by multidisciplinary efforts, will find much to ponder in this volume. Health services research raises a mixture of social, economic, institutional, and medical questions, and the methods for dealing with them are drawn from many disciplines. Well-formulated statements and assessments of the knowledge, experiences, and perspectives of experts in various fields offer a necessary building block for further research, and that is what we find in the chapters of *Cancer Care and Costs: DRGs and Beyond*.

By sponsoring the conference that led to this book, the American Cancer Society, California Division indicated its recognition that traditional concerns about community programs for cancer prevention, detection, treatment, and rehabilitation are affected by decisions in larger arenas—in this case, systems of reimbursement for care. In this volume, issues of cancer costs and public and private sources of reimbursement are joined with consequences, actual and speculative, for the functioning of sources of care and effective treatment and management of the patient. Explicit information is provided on the heavy social and health care costs of cancer, the changing burden of specific cancer sites as rates rise or fall, and the extent to which different sectors of health services are affected, with hospitals dominating the picture.

Since 1983, the elderly have been subject to the most extensive regulations for reimbursement of hospital care ever adopted by the federal government—the prospective payment system (PPS)—and this during a period of strong moves to deregulate other industries. The compelling reason was the need to moderate the escalation in hospital expenditures. The levers were economic incentives to reduce duration of stay and assessments of the appropriateness of admissions to the hospital; attention was to be given to quality of care.

In the past few years, significant reductions have occurred in hospital use, both generally and among cancer patients. Even if there were no further decreases, PPS could be viewed as an economic success story. Diagnosis-related groups may be modified or augmented by measures of severity of illness, resource-based relative value scales, or some other approach to increase equity in the system. In the long run, we may move more completely toward a capitated basis for reimbursement, which would cover inpatient and outpatient care. But there is no turning back to arrangements that do not exert pressure to control hospital utilization.

A mechanism for close scrutiny of the PPS for possible changes, large and small, is in place through the Prospective Payment Assessment Commission (ProPAC). We also have the Medicare Management Information System, a major resource for determining how PPS is functioning. However, there is more to be concerned about in PPS than the disbursement of funds and the impact of the system on hospital utilization. We still know too little about the influence of the system on the total care of cancer patients, the decisions by physicians and patients about where care is to be obtained, the changing relationships between hospitals and other sectors of care, and the quality of care reflected by morbidity, functional status, and mortality. These are not new issues; they have been discussed in general contexts, but they are sharpened when a specific set of diseases—in this case, cancer—is on the line.

This is made manifest in the cancer patient's ongoing need for extensive care from multiple types of providers and supportive services, which raises questions about access to and coordination of appropriate sources and levels of care. Concerns exist about possible lags in diffusion of technological advances and treatment, and about reluctance to engage in clinical research as a price for cost containment. If either concern became a far-reaching problem, the result would be a significant setback for the cancer field, in which achievement of goals for cancer control requires application of the results of years of cumulative research.

Further, and quite appropriately, the point is made in this book that we cannot allow our preoccupation with reimbursement problems related to PPS to detract from our attention to the promise of reducing cancer incidence and mortality through aggressive programs directed at personal health practices and early case findings.

Quality of care and, in particular, outcome of care is a pervasive issue in the book. Major efforts are needed to develop measures of outcome that include quality of life indicators. The results would, among other things, place in a more appropriate perspective the mortality figures for hospitals produced by the Health Care Financing Administration.

In the field of cancer, the highly charged issue of choices in the allocation of medical resources has special relevance, because complex and costly new technologies give promise for secondary prevention and, at the other end, for prolonging the lives of the severely ill. We may differ on how to define and resolve the implicit ethical issues, but the discussion of cancer costs would have been incomplete without the chapter on this topic.

Finally, one needs to question the effect of health care cost-containment measures on care for the economically disadvantaged in our population. The root of the question lies in the major disparities in cancer incidence and mortality rates between the poor and the rest of the population. These disparities are discussed in the final chapter of the volume and are accompanied by a challenge to allocate increased resources in an effort to change the situation.

Clearly, there is a long agenda for the health services researcher, and we should expect increased attention from investigators in this field to the general and specific issues that arise in the course of dealing with the economics of cancer care.

Sam Shapiro
Professor Emeritus
The Johns Hopkins University
School of Hygiene and Public Health
Department of Health Policy

Former Director, Health Services
Research and Development Center

Acknowledgments

This book examines recent changes in health care financing and their effects on cancer care and costs. Experts from a wide range of disciplines have contributed their perspectives on how to finance cancer care without compromising quality of care. The impetus for the volume was a conference sponsored in 1987 by the American Cancer Society (ACS), California Division. With considerable foresight, members of the society recognized that new interdisciplinary approaches were needed to address the complex issues surrounding DRGs, cancer care, and cost. The conference brought together leaders in medicine, public health, public policy, health insurance, medical economics, hospital administration, and cancer control to review and discuss how the changes in health care financing influence health care, its support systems, and patients with cancer and those at risk for cancer. The conference was planned through the efforts of a dedicated group of ACS volunteer and staff leaders. A special advisory committee provided planning, guidance, and support to identify key participants.

The editors wish to thank the planners and participants in that conference, particularly the members of the planning committee: Neil C. Andrews, Richard Bohannon, Maura C. Carroll, Paul Goldfarb, Lowell Irwin, David Collin, Helen Crothers, Glenn Hildebrand, Richard M. Scheffler, and Louise Torraco; and the members of the advisory committee: Robert Beck, Richard Bohannon, Adelbert Campbell, Joseph Hafey, Armand Hammer, John Hisserich, Robert Jamplis, Donald Kennedy, Kenneth Kizer, Bob Matsui, W. James Nethery, Martin Paley, Stanley Parry, C. D. Pruitt, Gary A. Ratkin, Dorothy P. Rice, Ruth Roemer, Leonard D. Schaeffer, Richard J. Steckel, and Charles H. White.

In addition, we would like to thank those who assisted with the book: Glenn Hildebrand at ACS for coordination and administration, George Schieber and his staff at the Health Care Financing

Administration (HCFA) for data support, and Lynn Maycock and
Barbara Martin for secretarial assistance.

Part I

Introductory
Framework

1 DRGs and the Financing of Cancer Care in the United States: New Estimates and New Issues

**Richard M. Scheffler and
Kathryn A. Phillips**

As health care spending in the United States increases dramatically, it continues to be a major focus of health policy and national debate. The share of the gross national product (GNP) consumed by health care rose from only 5.9 percent in 1965 to 11.1 percent in 1987 (Levit and Freeland 1988), the highest level in history and the highest of any major developed nation in the world (Schieber and Poullier 1986). During this period, public sector financing of health care increased dramatically. The percent of total health care costs borne by the public sector rose from approximately 26 percent in 1965 to 41 percent in 1987 (Levit and Freeland 1988), due primarily to the introduction and expansion of the Medicare and Medicaid programs. The Medicare program paid for 17 percent of all national health care expenditures in 1987 (Levit and Freeland 1988).

The increase in the costs of health care to the public sector has brought forth efforts to control those costs. The prospective payment system (PPS) was enacted for the Medicare program in 1983. Its purpose is to provide economic incentives that encourage cost-conscious behavior among hospitals and to ensure high-quality inpatient care. Under the Medicare PPS, payment to hospitals is made at a predetermined rate for each discharge, according to the diagnosis-related group (DRG) in which the discharge is classified. Currently, outpatient hospital care (i.e., emergency room, outpatient clinics) is not covered under PPS.

The change from cost-based reimbursement to a prospective payment system represents a fundamental change in the role of the Medicare program within our health care system. Under PPS, the federal government sets hospital prices rather than financing the actual cost of the care provided. However, the impact of PPS on *cancer* care and cost has not been thoroughly and rigorously examined. Thus, *Cancer Care and Cost: DRGs and Beyond* examines a variety of issues relating to the way cancer care has been affected by these changes in our health care system.

Why are we so concerned about cancer care? Cancer is the second leading cause of death in the United States and it accounts for about one-fourth of all deaths (National Center for Health Statistics 1987). The total costs of cancer, discussed in Chapter 3, are estimated at $72.5 billion. There has been a steady rise in the age-adjusted national death rate from cancer (American Cancer Society 1988). Predictions have been made that cancer incidence will increase over the next 40 to 50 years, so that by the year 2030, the number of new cases of cancer will double (Janerich 1984). The potential impact on the Medicare program and society in general is enormous, since our population is aging and cancer is more common in older age groups. Medicare pays a large majority of the expenses for cancer care for the aged; the Third National Cancer Survey (Scotto and Chiazze 1976) found that Medicare paid expenses in nearly 88 percent of cancer cases in patients over the age of 65.

The impact of PPS on care of cancer patients is a significant health policy issue with six central questions:

1. What is the impact of PPS on the *cost* of cancer care?

2. What is the impact of PPS on *patterns* of cancer care?

3. What is the impact of PPS on cancer *research* and the development of new technology?

4. How good are DRGs as a *measurement* tool for cancer care?

5. What is the impact of PPS on the *quality* of cancer care?

6. What is the impact of PPS on cancer care in the *health care system* as a whole?

This book addresses these issues from many different perspectives. This introductory chapter provides a framework for addressing these questions and presents an overall analysis of the impact of PPS on the cost and patterns of cancer care, using new data from the Medicare program.

THE IMPACT OF PPS ON THE COST OF CANCER CARE

Since a major incentive behind the implementation of PPS was the control of costs, it is appropriate to begin with this issue. Despite the high costs of inpatient cancer care and the significance of those costs to the Medicare system, few researchers have looked at the impact of PPS on the cost of cancer care. This analysis may be the first systematic examination on a national level of the impact of PPS on cancer costs in the Medicare program.

Analyzing changes in costs of care is a tricky business. One difficulty is determining whether changes in costs are a result of the implementation of PPS or a result of other factors. These factors include changes in the quality of care or severity of illness, price of services used in the hospital, competition or other health care market forces, changes in medical technology, and state cost-control policies. It is also difficult to compare costs before and after the implementation of PPS, since hospitals have switched their measurement of costs to adjust from a retrospective (cost-based) system to a prospective (price-setting) system. Defining "costs" is another tricky issue. Costs of care can be defined as billed charges, charges covered by Medicare, the level of charges paid, or the actual costs of production.

A study conducted by Lion and Henderson (1987) provides data on the costs of cancer care under Medicare. They analyzed oncology discharges from the 1984 Medicare Provider and Analysis Review (MEDPAR) file. Their research projected that the leading 15 sites of cancer accounted for over 75 percent of the total oncology discharges under Medicare. These 15 cancer sites generated $3.8 billion in charges. The most resource-intensive primary sites of cancer were cancers of the lung ($791 million), colon ($742 million), prostate ($418 million), breast ($341 million), and rectum ($317 million). While discharges with a primary diagnosis of cancer accounted for only 9.6 percent of Medicare discharges in those over age 65, the percent of the cost of cancer care is slightly higher (11.4 percent of the $45.5 billion spent for those over 65 for general hospital inpatient care in 1984).

The implementation of PPS and the rising costs of cancer care have made hospital administrators and staff more conscious of costs. One result has been an increased emphasis on "product line management" of oncology services. "Product line management" is an approach borrowed from business practices that uses cost data to determine DRG "winners and losers." Hospitals can see which "products" are "winners" (payments are greater than actual costs) and which are "losers" (payments are less than actual costs).

The Association of Community Cancer Centers (ACCC), whose member institutions are responsible for the management of one of every four new cancer cases in the United States (Rice 1986), has done some interesting work on DRG winners and losers. Based on 1985 data from over 20 hospitals of 300 beds or more, ACCC found that 15 cancer DRGs accounted for over 65 percent of all cancer inpatient discharges. Using data from 13,640 cancer discharges, there were $54.9 million generated in charges, $45.2 million in reimbursements, and approximately $42.8 million in estimated costs. These data suggest that cancer as a total product line may be a marginal winner on a cost basis. They also identified DRG winners (those with the highest margin above costs) and losers (those with the greatest loss). The top two winners were DRG 395, Red Blood Cell Disorders Age > 18 ($403,649 above cost on 779 discharges), and DRG 172, Digestive Malignancy Age > 70 and/or Complicating Conditions ($382,103 above cost on 553 discharges). The top two losers were DRG 410, Chemotherapy ($825,384 below cost on 1,372 discharges), and DRG 345, Other Male Reproductive System Operating Room Procedures except Malignancy ($812,042 below cost on 42 discharges).

This analysis is preliminary but quite suggestive. However, the important point is that this type of analysis (of winners and losers) is being conducted. The prospective payment system has changed incentives so that hospitals and cancer centers will want more DRG winners and fewer DRG losers. This generates real concern over the quality of treatment for cancer patients in the DRG loser category. Will hospitals reduce the quality and cost of DRG losers? Alternatively, will hospitals design policies to attract DRG winners? These are serious issues that require up-to-date answers and constant monitoring.

THE IMPACT OF PPS ON PATTERNS OF CANCER CARE

The prospective payment system changes the economic incentives for hospitals in providing cancer care. These incentives may affect patterns of care, including the mix of inpatient and outpatient care, the average length of stay for inpatient care, the types of patients that different facilities attempt to attract, the types and mix of services provided, and staffing patterns within the hospital.

Numerous studies have been conducted on the impact of PPS on overall hospital admissions and length of stay for inpatient care. Although causality cannot be directly determined, it is clear that major changes have taken place in the number of admissions and length of stay since the introduction of PPS. One of the most striking findings has been the decline in the number of admissions and discharges for all diagnoses (Guterman et al. 1988). Guterman et al. found that, in the first three years under PPS, admissions fell by a total of 11.3 percent and admissions per Medicare enrollee by 15.9 percent. There was a similar decline in the rate of discharges.

Most health policy experts did not foresee this decline in admissions. It appears to be the result of a combination of factors, including the rapid increase in outpatient hospital visits and technological changes that permit many procedures to be performed in outpatient settings. It is also likely that not including outpatient services under PPS helped to increase the substitution of outpatient services for inpatient services. Outpatient hospital services continue to be reimbursed using the cost-based system that was in effect prior to PPS.

The decline in length of stay under PPS was predicted by health policy experts (Guterman et al. 1988; U.S. Department of Health and Human Services 1987). Guterman et al. found that the average length of stay decreased 17 percent after the implementation of PPS. Hospitals have an incentive to reduce lengths of stay given the fixed payment for each admission; however, the size and speed of the decrease in length of stay was still surprising.

In addition to the aggregate numbers that show declines in admissions, discharges, and lengths of stay, there is anecdotal evidence that patterns of care are changing due to the implementation of PPS. For example, DRG 410, Chemotherapy, has been under-reimbursed (DRG payments do not cover cost). This underpayment may create a powerful incentive to use chemotherapy in less than optimal ways for patient treatment.[1] Anecdotal evidence suggests, for instance, that approximate dosages are reduced to permit the therapy to be given on an outpatient basis outside the strictures of PPS. Similarly, there is a marked disincentive to use infusion therapy—a process by which chemotherapeutic drugs are introduced slowly over an extended period of time—if it results in patient stays beyond the average length of stay for the chemotherapy DRG (Mortenson and Yarbro 1985).

The first two questions we have addressed—What is the impact of PPS on the *costs* of cancer care? What is the impact of PPS on *patterns* of cancer care?—are critical ones. However, since there is very little data available on these questions with specific relevance for cancer care, we obtained data from the Health Care Financing Administration (HCFA) on the costs and patterns of cancer care between 1983 and 1986. These data have not been analyzed previously, and they provide new and interesting insights into the impact of PPS on cancer care.

Data

The Health Care Financing Administration provided data from the hospital Medicare Provider Analysis and Review inpatient-stay record file for 1983–86.[2] This file is a 20 percent sample of Medicare stays and is generated by linking information from three HCFA master program files: the utilization bill file, the health insurance entitlement file, and the provider of services file. Cancer cases were identified by major diagnosis group, using the International Classification of Diseases (ICD) coding for neoplasms (ICD codes 140–234 except 209–229).[3] Comparisons were made between neoplasm ICDs and other diagnoses for number of discharges,[4] amount of charges, and lengths of stay. Charges for the most common cancers (lung, breast, colon, and prostate), accounting for 40 percent of inpatient neoplasm charges to Medicare, were separately identified.

Data were also broken down by whether or not the hospital was covered by PPS at the time the charge was submitted. According to the data, only 4 percent of charges in 1983 were in hospitals under PPS, but by 1986, 93 percent of charges were in hospitals covered by PPS. Those not covered in 1986 were cancer cases treated in cancer centers, which are not covered by PPS.

It is important to recognize the limitations of the data in attributing causation. As Richard J. Steckel discusses in Chapter 13, some cancer research centers have been excluded from PPS, so including them in the data makes it more difficult to attribute changes directly to the implementation of PPS. Furthermore, changes in cancer costs may be a result of many factors other than PPS, including changes in treatment protocols, regulatory efforts by states or the private sector to control the costs of health care, and changes in medical technology. Despite these limitations, these data can provide insights and identify specific issues for further research.

Findings

Number of discharges. Our findings for neoplasms mirror the general trend of a decline in the numbers of discharges, although our data indicate that the number of discharges for neoplasms declined at a more rapid rate than other diagnoses. Discharges for neoplasms fell 18 percent (890,035 discharges in 1983 to 730,280 discharges in 1986) versus 12.5 percent for other diagnoses (9,353,250 discharges in 1983 to 8,187,365 discharges in 1986 (See Table 1.1). Figure 1.1 illustrates this decline. When the data are adjusted for the number of Medicare enrollees,[5] the trend of declining discharges increases; discharges for neoplasms fell 20.7 percent and discharges for other diagnoses fell 17.4 percent.

Most of this decline was between 1983 and 1985. From 1985 to 1986 neoplasms declined only 2.6 percent as compared to 9.5 percent and 6.9 percent for 1984 – 85 and 1983 – 84, respectively. Other diagnoses showed virtually no decline from 1985 to 1986. Thus, we observe that the decline in discharges, which appears to be due to PPS, is "leveling off" for neoplasms and other diagnoses.

It is interesting to note the variability of the decline by type of cancer, particularly lung and colon cancer. Lung cancer discharges fell by 26.3 percent (126,135 to 92,925), while colon cancer discharges fell by only 3.4 percent (71,640 to 69,180) (see Table 1.2).

Length of stay. Our findings show that the average length of stay for neoplasms has been declining, although the rate of decline for neoplasms has been slower than the rate for other diagnoses. The average length of stay for neoplasms declined 9.7 percent (from 11.8 days in 1983 to 10.6 days in 1986) versus 12.1 percent for other diagnoses (from 9.7 days in 1983 to 8.5 days in 1986) (see Table 1.3). This decline is illustrated by Figure 1.2.

The finding by Guterman et al. (1988) of a leveling off of the decline in length of stay was also found with neoplasms; in the period 1985 – 86, the length of stay for neoplasms fell only 1.2

Table 1.1: Number of Medicare Discharges, 1983–86 (in thousands)

	1983	1984	Percent Change	1985	Percent Change	1986	Percent Change	Total Percent Change	Total Percent Change per Medicare Enrollee[a]
Neoplasms	890	828	-6.9%	750	-9.5%	730	-2.6%	-18.0	-20.7
Other diagnoses	9,353	8,877	-5.1	8,168	-8.0	8,156	-0.23	-12.5	-17.4

Source: Unpublished data, Health Care Financing Administration, 1988.
Note: Yearly totals are rounded to nearest 1,000. Percent changes are based on totals before rounding.
[a]Figures were adjusted for the increase in Medicare enrollment from 30 million in 1983 to 31.7 million in 1986 (Health Care Financing Administration, Division of National Cost Estimates, 1987).

Figure 1.1: Number of Medicare Discharges, 1983 – 86

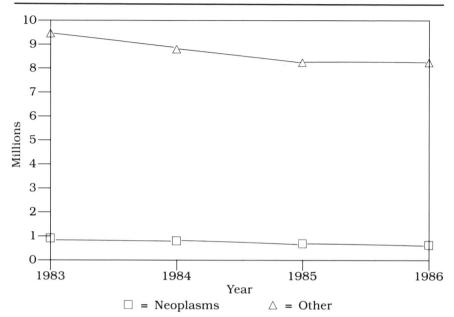

percent, from 10.65 to 10.64 days. Another interesting finding is that the length of stay for neoplasms was higher than for other diagnoses in 1983 (11.8 days versus 9.7 days) and has stayed higher (in 1986, 10.6 days versus 8.5 days).

The variability in discharges by type of cancer is also evident for length of stay. Lengths of stay for breast cancer and prostate cancer fell the most (33.3 percent and 22.9 percent, respectively) while lung cancer and colon cancer fell the least (7.5 percent and 8.5 percent, respectively) (see Table 1.4).

Costs. Total charges to Medicare for neoplasms relative to total charges for all diagnoses have remained steady at approximately 10 percent. Total charges for neoplasms have also increased at approximately the same rate as other diagnoses, rising an average of 28.7 percent per discharge (from $5,837 in 1983 to $7,513 in 1986) and 42.5 percent per day (from $496 in 1983 to $706 in 1986). Total charges for other diagnoses rose an average of 24.7 percent per discharge (from $4,624 in 1983 to $5,763 in 1986) and

Table 1.2: Number of Medicare Discharges by Cancer Site, 1983–86 (in thousands)

	1983	1984	Percent Change	1985	Percent Change	1986	Percent Change	Total Percent Change
Breast	67	60	−10.0%	57	−4.9%	59	3.8%	−11.1%
Lung	126	111	−11.7	96	−13.9	93	−3.2	−26.3
Prostate	94	89	−5.2	80	−10.0	81	1.1	−13.7
Colon	72	71	−1.5	69	−2.5	69	0.61	−3.4

Note: Yearly totals are rounded to nearest 1,000. Percent changes are based on totals before rounding.

Table 1.3: Average Length of Stay for Medicare Patients, 1983–86 (in days)

	1983	1984	Percent Change	1985	Percent Change	1986	Percent Change	Total Percent Change
Neoplasms	11.77	10.96	– 6.9%	10.65	– 2.8%	10.64	– 1.2%	– 9.7%
Other diagnoses	9.68	8.67	– 10.4	8.47	– 2.3	8.51	– 0.5	– 12.1

Figure 1.2: Average Length of Stay for Medicare Patients,
1983 – 86

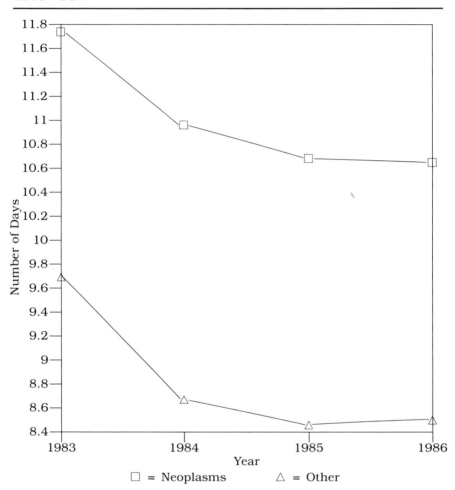

□ = Neoplasms   △ = Other

41.8 percent per day (from $478 in 1983 to $677 in 1986) (see
Table 1.5). These increases are shown in Figures 1.3 and 1.4. The
similarity in the increases per discharge for neoplasms and other
diagnoses is quite interesting since the drop in lengths of stay for
neoplasms has been slower than for other diagnoses.

The variability between types of cancer in average total
charges per discharge is large. The average charge per discharge
declined 2.7 percent for breast cancer, while it rose 36.4 percent

Table 1.4: Average Length of Stay by Cancer Site for Medicare Patients, 1983–86 (in days)

	1983	1984	Percent Change	1985	Percent Change	1986	Percent Change	Total Percent Change
Breast	10.12	8.61	−14.9%	7.38	−14.3%	6.75	−8.5%	−33.3%
Lung	11.83	10.98	−7.2	10.89	−0.8	10.94	0.5	−7.5
Prostate	9.67	8.56	−11.5	7.84	−8.4	7.46	−4.9	−22.9
Colon	15.78	15.03	−4.8	14.42	−4.1	14.44	0.1	−8.5

Table 1.5: Average Charges to Medicare, 1983–86 (in dollars)

	1983	1984		1985		1986		
	Per Discharge	Per Discharge	Percent Change	Per Discharge	Percent Change	Per Discharge	Percent Change	Total Percent Change
Neoplasms	$5,837	$6,141	5.2%	$6,781	10.4%	$7,513	10.8%	28.7%
Other diagnoses	4,624	4,718	2.0	5,184	9.9	5,763	11.2	24.7

	1983	1984		1985		1986		
	Per Day	Per Day	Percent Change	Per Day	Percent Change	Per Day	Percent Change	Total Percent Change
Neoplasms	$496	$560	13.1%	$637	13.6%	$706	10.9%	42.5%
Other diagnoses	478	544	13.9	612	12.5	677	10.7	41.8

Figure 1.3: Average Charge to Medicare per Discharge,
1983 – 86 (in dollars)

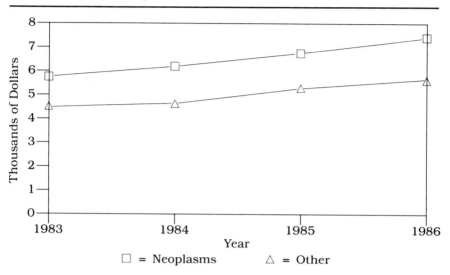

Figure 1.4: Average Charge to Medicare per Day,
1983 – 86 (in dollars)

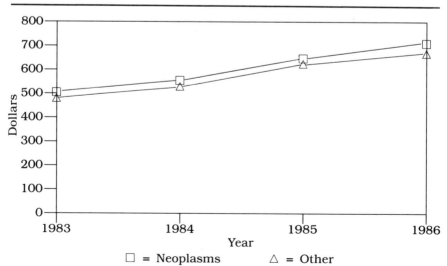

Table 1.6: Average Charges to Medicare per Discharge and per Day by Cancer Site, 1983–86 (in dollars)

	1983	1984		1985		1986		
	Per Discharge	Per Discharge	Percent Change	Per Discharge	Percent Change	Per Discharge	Percent Change	Total Percent Change
Breast	$4,482	$4,312	-3.8%	$4,305	-0.2%	$4,363	1.3%	-2.7%
Lung	5,980	6,353	6.2	7,196	13.3	8,156	13.3	36.4
Prostate	4,341	4,336	-0.1	4,533	4.6	4,784	5.5	10.2
Colon	8,528	9,211	8.0	10,018	8.8	11,085	10.7	30.0

	1983	1984		1985		1986		
	Per Day	Per Day	Percent Change	Per Day	Percent Change	Per Day	Percent Change	Total Percent Change
Breast	$443	$501	13.2%	$583	16.4%	$647	11.0%	46.1%
Lung	505	578	14.4	661	14.3	746	12.8	47.5
Prostate	449	506	12.8	578	14.7	642	11.0	42.9
Colon	541	613	13.3	695	13.4	768	10.5	42.0

for lung cancer during the period 1983 – 86. However, average charges per day rose approximately the same amount (greater than 40 percent) for the four types of cancer (see Table 1.6).

In conclusion, we observe that PPS has had an important impact on cancer care in the Medicare program. Cancer discharges dropped more dramatically than other discharges, but the decline in average length of stay was smaller. The declines in cancer discharges and lengths of stay are both leveling off in a fashion similar to noncancer cases. The vast differences between cancer sites, in terms of discharges and lengths of stay, warrant further explanation and monitoring. Outpatient hospital treatment and treatment in physician offices may explain some of these differences. Another explanation may be changes in treatments, such as the trend toward less radical treatments for breast cancer. We found that increases in charges per day and per admission were similar for neoplasms and other diagnoses over the 1983 – 86 period.

CANCER RESEARCH AND THE DEVELOPMENT OF NEW TECHNOLOGY

Cancer treatment is constantly evolving as different combinations and new applications of existing therapies, as well as the development of new therapies, improve the state of oncological practice. In many instances, the best treatment for the patient will involve the use of new procedures that differ from those employed with other patients at earlier times. Thus, in many cases, the current cost of treatment will be more than the historical costs (Mortenson and Yarbro 1985). These characteristics of cancer treatment have led to concerns that a prospective reimbursement system will not adequately reimburse for new treatments, research, and new technology.

Although there is little direct evidence on this issue, several researchers have addressed the potential impact of PPS on cancer research and innovation. Mortenson (1986) postulated that PPS will be a disincentive for hospitals to participate in clinical trials, since patients in the trials may have longer lengths of stay. Under the reimbursement system, Medicare did not specifically pay for clinical research, but the greatest part of research expenses were covered because reimbursement was made without reference to length of stay. He also suggested that, since recent cancer care innovations may not be accounted for in the reimbursement computations for DRGs, PPS may discourage the use of such innovations. This is an especially critical problem in oncology where innovations in cancer care may require new technical resources, such as implantable pumps, or more extensive support and longer hospitalization.

DRGs AS A MEASUREMENT TOOL FOR CANCER CARE

This issue is extremely important given the variation in severity of illness of patients within DRGs. Horn and Sharkey (1986) examined case mix and financial data for 4,390 cases in 40 cancer-related DRGs from 15 hospitals. The observed heterogeneity of severity of illness within DRGs could have major financial effects on hospitals, since not all hospitals' cancer patients exhibit the same distribution of severity of illness. The hospitals with cancer centers treated proportionately more of the severely ill patients than did the noncancer centers. Therefore, prospective payment based on fixed DRG payments could be very inequitable to these and other institutions that attract the severely ill patients, with the potential long-term consequences of closure of specialty treatment centers, refusal to admit certain patients, or reduction in quality of care.

They also found that there is a great deal of variation in cost per case for patients classified into the 40 cancer-related DRGs. DRGs explained about 15 percent of the variation in cost per case data in their data set. The explanatory power increased to 58.4 percent when DRGs were subdivided by severity of illness and procedure type.

More recent research by Lion and Henderson (1987) has continued to examine the case mix of oncology care. Their preliminary findings indicate that, for lung cancer, the most common DRGs—medical treatment of malignant lung neoplasms, chemotherapy for lung cancer, and major chest procedures—have significantly different mean charges and better coefficients of variation than the overall mean and coefficients of variation for all Medicare discharges with a diagnosis of neoplasms of the lung as the primary site of cancer. The conclusion in the case of this leading cancer, therefore, is that the DRGs actually do improve the reimbursement for lung cancer. The same situation prevails for breast cancer and, to a lesser extent, for colon, prostate, and malignant lymphoma. Lion and Henderson have continued to research the question of whether the DRGs themselves could be further improved if those DRGs containing the most common cancers are modified in more substantial detail.

THE IMPACT OF PPS ON THE QUALITY OF CANCER CARE

A fundamental issue concerning PPS is its impact on the quality of care. There are many ways to frame the quality debate. The Health Care Financing Administration has been tracking mortality rates and readmission rates to measure changes in quality of care. To date, the data do not suggest that PPS has had a great impact on either mortality or readmission rates. Mortality rates have increased, but these increases appear to be explainable by the changing diagnostic mix of hospitalized patients (Guterman et al. 1988). Yet these aggregate figures do not tell the complete story about quality of care, an issue addressed by several authors in this book (see Part IV).

PPS AND CANCER CARE IN THE HEALTH CARE SYSTEM AS A WHOLE

The implementation of PPS is just one part of the larger trend toward cost containment in our health care system. Four specific developments are viewed as the foundations of cost containment: the introduction of PPS, the proliferation of new forms of prepaid health care delivery, the increasing supply of physicians, and the growth of for-profit health care enterprises (Ginzberg 1987). These developments have undoubtedly affected cancer care in many ways. One area of particular interest for cancer care and costs is the impact of cost containment on prevention. Bailar and Smith (1986) report that age-adjusted mortality rates from cancer have shown a slow and steady increase over several decades, and they argue that prevention is the key to reducing the toll from cancer. Yet, it remains to be seen whether PPS and other attempts at cost containment will encourage or discourage the provision of preventive services. On the one hand, the Medicare program has added coverage of mammograms beginning in 1990. On the other hand, PPS may have changed the pattern of care for cancer patients in a direction that is economically more acceptable but less agreeable to patients and providers. The possible trade-offs between cost containment and the prevention and appropriate treatment of cancer patients constitute the overriding theme of this book. We must not lose sight of the fact that savings to the Medicare program on inpatient treatment, which are attributed to PPS, may simply represent a shift to costs of outpatient hospital or physician care. We also need to consider the costs to cancer patients and their families that result from earlier discharges from the hospital.

CONCLUSION

We have addressed six important questions concerning the impact of PPS on cancer care and costs. These and other issues are discussed further in the remainder of this book. Only time and more research will tell us whether cost-containment programs such as PPS are successful, and whether they have hurt or helped our fight against cancer.

NOTES

1. In Chapter 4, Steven F. Jencks offers one explanation of why chemotherapy is under-reimbursed.
2. We are grateful to George Schieber and his staff at HCFA for providing the data and calculations we requested.
3. ICD coding gives a more comprehensive picture of cancer costs than DRG coding since surgical DRGs consist of noncancer as well as cancer cases.
4. Numbers of admissions were not available, but for the purposes of this trend analysis, admissions and discharges can be treated interchangeably.
5. The number of enrollees shows a small upward trend, from approximately 30 million in 1983, 30.5 million in 1984, 31.1 million in 1985, to 31.7 million in 1986. See Division of National Cost Estimates, Office of the Actuary, "National Health Expenditures, 1986 – 2000," *Health Care Financing Review* 8, no. 4 (August 1987).

REFERENCES

American Cancer Society. (1988). *Cancer Facts and Figures—1988.* New York: American Cancer Society.

Bailar, J. C., and Smith, E. M. (1986). "Progress Against Cancer?" *The New England Journal of Medicine* 314(19): 1226 – 32.

Ginzberg, E. (1987). "A Hard Look at Cost Containment." *The New England Journal of Medicine* 316(8): 1151 – 54.

Guterman, S.; Eggers, P. W.; Riley, G.; Greene, T. F.; and Terrell, S. A. (1988). "The First Three Years of Medicare Prospective Payment: An Overview." *Health Care Financing Review* 9(3): 67 – 77.

Horn, S. D., and Sharkey, P. D. (1986). "A Study of Patients in Cancer-Related DRGs." *Journal of Cancer Program Management* (November): 8 – 14.

Janerich, D. T. (1984). "Forecasting Cancer Trends to Optimize Control Strategies." *Journal of the National Cancer Institute* 72(6): 1317 – 21.

Levit, K., and Freeland, M. (1988). "National Medical Care Spending." *Health Affairs* 7(5): 124 – 36.

Lion, J., and Henderson, M. (1987). "A DRG-Based Case Mix Analysis of Oncology Care." Unpublished report, Brandeis University, Waltham, MD.

Mortenson, L. E. (1986). "Cancer Diagnosis Related Groups." In *Advances in Cancer Control: Health Care Financing and Research.* 149 – 54. New York: Alan R. Liss.

Mortenson, L. E., and Yarbro, J. W. (1985). *Cancer DRGs: A Comparative Report on the Key Cancer DRGs.* Rockville, MD: Association of Community Cancer Centers.

National Center for Health Statistics. (1987). "Advance Report of Final Mortality Statistics, 1985." *Monthly Vital Statistics Report* 34(13). DHHS Pub. No. (PHS) 87-1120. Washington, DC: U.S. Government Printing Office.

Rice, W. W. (1986). "Oncology and Product Line Management: Pitfalls in Practice." *Health Care Strategic Management* (October): 4 – 8.

Schieber, G. J., and Poullier, J. P. (1986). "International Health Care Spending." *Health Affairs* 5(3): 111 – 22.

Scotto, J., and Chiazze, L. (1976). *Third National Cancer Survey: Hospitalizations and Payments to Hospitals, Part A: Summary.* U.S. Department of Health, Education, and Welfare. DHEW Pub. No. (NIH) 76-1094. Washington, DC: U.S. Government Printing Office.

U.S. Department of Health and Human Services. (1987). *The Impact of the Medicare Hospital Prospective Payment System, 1985 Annual Report.* Report to Congress. HCFA Pub. No. 03251. Washington, DC: U.S. Government Printing Office.

2 Health Care Financing and Cancer Treatment: A Historical Overview

Neil C. Andrews

The cost of health care in the United States has risen to an unacceptably high level. The adverse effects have been felt in every sector of society. Businesses have raised prices to accommodate employee health benefits. The federal government has found that the cost of Medicare, Medicaid, and other health programs are exceeding predictions. The public has suddenly discovered that many of its members can no longer afford medical care. The response of government to the high cost of Medicare has been to substitute a prospective method of reimbursement for the retrospective method that was previously used to reimburse health care providers. The development and implementation of the DRG system of reimbursement has implications for cancer patients and for patterns of cancer care.

Simultaneously, an explosion of medical research and a transformation in health care delivery have elevated the science and practice of medicine to unanticipated levels of sophistication. Several factors can be identified as contributors to the explosive rise in the cost of health care: an increase in the number of physicians, physician specialization, an increase in the number of hospital beds, changes in patient expectations, governmental responses to perceived needs, technological advances, changes in the delivery of health care, inflation, and others.

THE PHYSICIAN POPULATION

In 1964, a total of 297,000 physicians practiced medicine in the United States (including 12,900 osteopathic physicians). The ratio of physicians to the population had remained constant since 1950, at about 150 per 100,000 (Clark 1967, 824).

Based on the assumption that the citizens of the United States were receiving inadequate health care as a result of a shortage of medical and other health professionals, the federal government passed the Health Professions Educational Assistance Act in 1963 (Sullivan 1967). During the next 15 years, classes in existing medical schools were expanded and new schools of medicine were established. In California, classes at the established schools of medicine were increased in size and three new schools of medicine were established by the University of California: at Davis, Los Angeles (Irvine), and San Diego. The immigration of many foreign physicians, plus programs to bring physicians educated in other countries to the United States for training, also increased the number of physicians in this country.

The total number of physicians in the United States in 1976 was 348,443 (American Medical Association 1977). By 1980, an estimated 426,300 doctors of medicine and 17,700 doctors of osteopathy were practicing medicine (Burton, Smith, and Nichols 1980, 78). In 1975, there were 42,194 nonfederal physicians who were actively practicing medicine in California, serving an estimated civilian population of 21,239,000—a ratio of 198.7 physicians to 100,000 persons (California Medical Association 1976). By 1985, the number of physicians had risen to 63,009 and the ratio to 239.3 per 100,000 people (California Medical Association 1987a).

In 1976, it was estimated that each new practicing physician resulted in an increase of $250,000 in the annual cost of medical care to society (Reinhardt 1976). Ten years later, the California Medical Association reported that the cost for each new physician entering practice was almost $475,000 (California Medical Association 1987b, 42).

Between 1950 and 1964, the number of general practitioners in the United States decreased from 101,000 to 67,000, while the number of specialists increased from 57,000 to 111,000 (Clark 1967, 825). By 1985, out of a total of 63,009 doctors practicing in California, 10,377 specialized in internal medicine, 15,421 in surgery, 3,022 in anesthesia, and 4,395 in psychiatry (California Medical Association 1987b, 3). Between December 1973 and

December 1983, the charges for physician services increased by 159 percent (California Medical Association 1984). The increase in the number of physicians, the increase in the number of specialists, and the increase in physicians' income undoubtedly contributed to the increased cost of health care.

PAYMENT SYSTEMS

As the characteristics of the physician population were changing, so were the patterns of care for patients. During the depression, when many people were unemployed, patients reimbursed physicians with cash, services, or goods. However, bartering was not acceptable for payment of hospital costs. Patients who were unable to pay any or all of their hospital bills were accommodated by the hospital, which used cost shifting to make up the deficit. Other patients paid inflated bills to support these costs, and additional funds came from the public sector, government, and philanthropists.

In 1929, Blue Cross insurance was started with Baylor Medical School to provide direct payment to participating hospitals for most charges incurred by patients who were policyholders. Blue Shield was established separately to pay surgical fees (Burton, Smith, and Nichols 1980, 106). Both plans expanded rapidly. In the 1930s, Kaiser-Permanente established a prepaid health plan that became the prototype for the health maintenance organization (Burton, Smith, and Nichols 1980, 109). Although it originated in California, this plan expanded to other states during the 1940s to cover Kaiser shipbuilding employees. Employers became increasingly involved in the payment of insurance premiums for health care. This was particularly true during World War II, when wages were fixed but benefits were not. In addition to higher wages, unions demanded fringe benefits, including health insurance, to improve the status of their members.

FEDERAL LEGISLATION

The federal government had been involved in health care as early as 1798, when Congress established the Marine Hospital Service for the care of sick and disabled seamen. The first hospital was established in Boston and others were opened at principal ports and waterways during the next few years. The Marine Hospital Service was incorporated into the new U.S. Public Health Service in 1912. A laboratory established at the Staten Island Marine Hospital in 1887, and moved to Washington in 1891, was the forerunner of the National Institutes of Health (Burton, Smith, and Nichols 1980, 47).

Congress created the Social Security program in 1935 to provide old age and survivor's insurance, contributions to state unemployment insurance programs, and assistance for the elderly. Later, the federal government attempted to provide health care to its older citizens through programs that required both federal and state support, such as the Kerr-Mills Act. This program was unsuccessful because many states failed to allocate the necessary funds to support it (Burton, Smith, and Nichols 1980, 111).

By 1964, the population of the United States had increased to 190,723,000 and health and medical care expenditures totaled $35,401,000 (Klarman 1967, 769). In 1965, legislation established Title XVIII (Medicare) and Title XIX (Medicaid). These programs were expanded in 1972 to include disabled beneficiaries of the Social Security and Railroad Retirement programs and persons requiring dialysis or kidney transplantation for end-stage renal disease (Burton, Smith, and Nichols 1980, 112–17).

By 1975, health care expenditures had risen to $131 billion or 8.6 percent of the gross national product, and Joseph Califano, then Secretary of the Department of Health, Education, and Welfare, estimated that this cost would rise to $368 billion or 10.2 percent of the GNP by 1984. He also estimated that 83 million Americans, 40 percent of the population, lacked insurance protection against very large medical bills (Califano 1979).

In 1977, 71 percent of the U.S. population had some form of insurance, 10 percent were covered by Medicare, 8 percent by Medicaid, 3.5 percent by the military, 1 percent by the Veterans Administration, and 0.5 percent by other plans; and 6 percent had no insurance (Sudovar and Sullivan 1980). Since the cost of medical care was paid by third parties, the patients who were covered by these plans became more and more demanding. Hospitalization was requested and received, sophisticated diagnostic studies were requested and performed, referrals to specialists were requested and granted. The concept of medical care as an inherent right of citizenship was accepted as fact.

Medicaid, which was enacted at the same time as Medicare, cost $2.5 billion in 1967 (Cooper, Worthington, and McGee 1976). By 1976, the cost of this program had risen to $15.3 billion (Gibson and Mueller 1977). Congress and the states moved to reduce these expenditures by tightening eligibility requirements and curtailing benefits.

MEDI-CAL

In California, Medicaid was known as Medi-Cal. Initially, its aim was to provide equal access to health care for all citizens of California. However, by August 1967, it was necessary to cut back expenditure to avoid potentially severe budget deficits. Regulations were passed to reduce the number of eligible recipients as well as the benefits provided; yet, the program still remained costly. In 1981, the state legislature cut $200 million from the $4 billion in the Medi-Cal budget. Reimbursements to hospitals and physicians were reduced to levels below those paid by other forms of insurance. In 1982, the California legislature authorized the governor to appoint a Medi-Cal "czar" whose responsibility was to negotiate with hospitals for the most favorable reimbursement rates for treatment of Medi-Cal patients. These negotiations were required to be conducted in absolute secrecy so that other hospitals in the community would not have an advantage in their negotiations with the czar. This resulted in agreements with hospitals that reduced their reimbursements to between 5 and 20 percent below normal payments. In addition, the legislature allowed third-party payers to negotiate prepaid rates with both hospitals and doctors (Iglehart 1984).

As an additional cost-cutting measure, the legislature authorized the transfer of responsibility for the medically indigent patient from Medi-Cal to the county. This resulted in inadequate health care for many poor and medically indigent persons.

Medi-Cal expenditures were estimated to have decreased by $470 million during the fiscal year 1983 – 84. Medi-Cal reimbursements to hospitals dropped from 83.2 percent to 73.2 percent of costs between 1982 and 1986 (California Association of Hospitals and Health Systems 1987). For the period July – September 1988, physician reimbursement by Medi-Cal for all procedure codes was 41 percent of reasonable and customary fees (California Department of Health Services 1988).

HOSPITAL EXPANSION AND ESCALATING COSTS

In the mid-1940s, health care was perceived to be inadequate in many areas of the United States, particularly in the inner cities and in rural communities. The government responded by establishing the Hill-Burton program in 1946. This legislation authorized grants to states to construct and equip public and voluntary, nonprofit, general, and other hospitals (Burton, Smith, and Nichols 1980, 86). The original law required each state to establish a planning mechanism for evaluating the status of present and future hospitals. In 1964, an amendment was added specifying that any hospital that accepted Hill-Burton funds could not discriminate against patients on the basis of race, color, or national origin. In addition, any hospital that accepted Hill-Burton funds was obligated to provide, on an annual basis, a dollar volume of uncompensated services equal to the lesser of 3 percent of operating costs (minus Medicaid and Medicare reimbursements) or 10 percent of the amount of federal assistance it received, adjusted for inflation over a 20-year period (U.S. Department of Health and Human Services 1986).

Between 1946 and 1975, nearly 500,000 acute care and long-term care hospital beds were added. The federal share of $4.1 billion was matched by $10.4 billion contributed by states and local interests (Clark 1981, 698).

Insurance companies, Medicare, and, to a lesser extent, Medicaid established a system through which hospitals were reimbursed according to their expenditures. Thus, when a hospital increased its expenditures, its income also increased. This created an ideal climate for the hospital to expand its services, to institute new technologies, to purchase new equipment, and to increase wages for employees.

Between December 1973 and December 1983, hospital room charges and drug costs increased 245.2 percent and 120.8 percent, respectively (California Medical Association 1984). In 1981 alone, hospital costs increased 17.9 percent to $12.2 billion, in contrast to food prices, which rose only 5.3 percent, and housing, which rose by 11.1 percent (Melia et al. 1983). However, there was a negative side to the income equation. Hospitals lost income from bad debts, charity care, and below-standard reimbursement from some payers. In California, these losses have been estimated to be 7.5 percent of total charges, increasing from $895 million in 1982 to a projected $1.5 billion for 1986 ($900 million in bad debts and charity care, and $600 million in Medi-Cal shortfalls) (Roffers 1986).

During 1982, hospitals in the United States provided $6.2 billion worth of uncompensated care, of which $1.7 billion went to charity cases. The medically underserved patients who were treated included 30 to 35 million unsponsored Americans and 21 to 26 million underinsured Americans. Sixty-five percent of the uninsured were either working or dependent upon an employed

person. Many entered this category after the recession of 1981 – 82
when many manufacturing jobs were replaced by service jobs.
Others were divorced or widowed women, the elderly, the chroni-
cally ill, those with preexisting illnesses who were unable to obtain
health insurance, the disabled who were not disabled enough to
qualify for Medicaid, and the victims of compromised health
(Friedman 1986). The American Hospital Association has estimated that 55.4 percent of charity care is provided by public hospitals, 44.1 percent by private nonprofit hospitals, and 0.5 percent
by investor-owned hospitals (Bazzoli 1985).

THE DEVELOPMENT OF CANCER TREATMENTS

The essentials of cancer treatment are surgery, radiation therapy,
and chemotherapy. In the late 1800s, with radiology in its infancy,
surgery emerged as the method of choice for the treatment of cancer. Although there were other great surgeons, few had the impact
of William Stewart Halsted of Johns Hopkins University. In 1891,
he described the technique of radical mastectomy for cancer of the
breast and established the standard treatment for this disease for
the next 100 years (Holleb and Randers-Pehrson 1987, 109 – 11;
Haagensen 1971, 411). His teachings regarding en-bloc removal of
the cancer, with due regard to lymphatic drainage of the breast
and the avoidance of wound contamination by loose cancer cells,
became the standards that would be incorporated into all forms of
cancer surgery.

Some surgeons, with the freedom allowed by improved anesthesia, blood products, antibiotics, and improved understanding
of the biochemical and physiologic effects of surgical therapy on
the human body, attempted to extend the range of surgery to the
complete removal of all cancer cells in advanced disease. However,
procedures such as hemipelvectomies and quarterectomies
resulted in low ratios of cures to treatment and were, for the most
part, discontinued. Since then, the pendulum has swung toward a
reduction in the extent of surgery and an emphasis upon adjuvant
therapy. Radiation therapy has changed markedly during the
twentieth century. As an understanding of this modality has
developed, techniques have been refined for delivering radiation,
and new sources of radiation energy have been developed.

Prior to World War II, only a few drugs were available for the
treatment of specific diseases (Burton, Smith, and Nichols 1980,

344, 350). Prior to World War I, those drugs included salversan, quinine, and Prontosil. A monumental study by Paul Ehrlich resulted in the synthesis of the agent that he called "606" (because it was the 606th arsenical drug that he had developed), which was most useful in the treatment of syphilis in both animals and humans (Marquardt 1951). Quinine extracted from the bark of the cinchona tree had been a familiar treatment for malaria since 1633 (Goodman and Gilman 1985, 1062). Prontosil, an azo dye containing the sulfonamide group, was first used for streptococcal infections by Foerster in 1933. This was followed by the study and use of sulfanilamide and other sulfa drugs in the pre-penicillin period (Goodman and Gilman 1985, 1113).

The shortage of quinine after the Japanese invasion of the Dutch East Indies stimulated an extensive program of research into therapy for malaria. This research, conducted between 1941 and 1945, was supported mainly by the Committee on Medical Research of the Office of Scientific Research and Development. The program involved industrial firms, the U.S. Army, and the Public Health Service (Marshall 1964).

In 1946, a report was published regarding the use of nitrogen mustards in malignancies of the lymphatic tissue. These chemicals had been under investigation since 1942 for their possible value in the treatment of neoplasms (Gilman and Philips 1946). Interest in the use of nitrogen mustard to treat malignancies had been motivated by the observation that, several days after exposure to mustard gas, military personnel developed bronchopneumonia and leukopenia, in addition to the toxicity to the skin and eyes. At autopsy, dissolution of the lymphoid tissue, gastrointestinal ulceration, and depression of the bone marrow were found (Krumbharr and Krumbharr 1919).

The study of nitrogen mustard and its chemical relatives was supported by a contract between Yale University and the United States Office of Scientific Research and Development. This investigation was assigned to Louis S. Goodman and Alfred Gilman, who were joined by Frederick Philips and Roberta Allen (Gilman 1963). Studies of the pharmacology of these agents were done in rabbits, rats, and cats (Hunt and Philips 1949). Thomas Dougherty, a colleague in the Department of Anatomy, gave nitrogen mustard to a single mouse with an advanced lymphoma (Gilman 1963). Complete regression of the tumor occurred and persisted for one month. After additional studies on mice with transplanted lymphoma, the investigational use of this agent was initiated in the treatment of human malignant disease (Calabresi and Parks 1975).

The first clinical trial of nitrogen mustard was conducted at Yale University by Gilman, Goodman, Dougherty, and Lindskog in 1942 (Gilman 1963). The patient had a malignant lymphoma that had become radioresistant. He was given nitrogen mustard intravenously for ten days. Within 48 hours, the tumor masses softened, and by the fourth day, signs and symptoms of the disease were abating. By the tenth day, cervical lymph nodes could no longer be palpated; by the fourteenth day, enlarged axillary lymph nodes were no longer apparent. The tumor recurred after one month and a second course of nitrogen mustard was given with only transient response. The patient died after a third course of nitrogen mustard was administered three months after the initial treatment, but the tumor burden was relatively small. At the time of death, the patient had bone marrow depression and thrombopenia (Gilman 1963; Goodman et al. 1946).

In 1948, researchers reported on the use of the folic acid antagonist, aminopterin, in the treatment of children with acute leukemia (Farber et al. 1948).

Screening programs to identify chemical agents that are effective against cancer were established at the Sloan-Kettering Institute, the National Cancer Institute, the Children's Cancer Research Foundation, the Southern Research Institute, the Chester Beatty Research Institute in London, the Cancer Institute in Moscow, and the University of Tokyo. The National Cancer Institute established the Cancer Chemotherapy National Service Center (CCNSC) to supervise the screening of potential cancer drugs (Goldin and Carter 1973).

In 1955, Cruz, McDonald, and Cole observed that when a suspension of Walker 256 cells was injected into the portal vein of Sprague-Dawley rats, followed after one minute by an injection of nitrogen mustard, the number of metastatic lesions in the liver at four weeks fell to 19.4 percent of the number that developed without the nitrogen mustard injection (Cruz, McDonald, and Cole 1956).

In 1956, a clinical study of breast cancer in patients under 70 yeas old was initiated at the University of Illinois to test the effectiveness of adjuvant anticancer chemotherapy after radical mastectomy. Seventy-eight control patients received no treatment and seventy-eight patients were given nitrogen mustard both immediately following surgery and on the following two days. Recurrences developed in 50 percent of the control patients and in only 39.7 percent of those receiving nitrogen mustard (Mrazek 1970).

These and other observations led to the initiation in 1957 of the Surgical Adjuvant Chemotherapy Program, sponsored by the National Cancer Institute. This program was developed to statistically compare survivorship of cancer patients following surgical resection alone against a comparable group of patients who received an anticancer drug at the same time that the surgical procedure was performed. The rationale for the studies was that a small number of cancer cells left in the patient following surgery could result in recrudescence of the cancer at a later time. If these cells could be killed by a chemotherapeutic agent, recurrence could be prevented and survival rates increased (Moore, Ross, and Stiver 1963). Groups were formed to study the effects of chemotherapeutic agents given during and after surgery to patients with cancer of the breast, stomach, colon-rectum, ovary, urinary bladder, and lung. Similar studies were initiated by the Veterans Administration.

In the 1960s, many physicians who had been involved in the adjuvant chemotherapy trials were given an opportunity to participate in one of the established or newly formed clinical cooperative groups. These trials were conducted under the direction and support of the Cancer Chemotherapy National Service Center. Most of these groups consisted of investigators in universities with facilities to conduct clinical cancer research. The mission of these groups was to conduct protocol studies in humans of the hundreds of cancer chemotherapeutic agents that were effective in animal tumors. Most of the cooperative groups were supported by grants or contracts from the CCNSC (Zubrod et al. 1966).

The treatment of cancer has changed markedly during the latter part of the twentieth century. Surgery is no longer the only treatment available for cancer. Radiologic and medical oncology have achieved maturity, and both are now used adjunctively with surgery to improve survival rates for cancer patients. The rest of this book examines how DRGs and other cost-saving measures have affected cancer treatment, whether they have reduced the cost of cancer care, and whether patients who develop cancer in this new era will be able to obtain timely and appropriate treatment.

REFERENCES

American Medical Association. (1977). "Physician Master File." In *Preventive and Community Medicine*, 2nd ed., edited by D. W. Clark and B. MacMahon, 701. Boston: Little, Brown and Company, 1981.

Bazzoli, G. J. (1985). *Health Care for the Indigent: Literature Review and Research Agenda for the Future*. Chicago: American Hospital Publishing.

Burton, L. E.; Smith, H. H.; and Nichols, A. W. (1980). *Public Health and Community Medicine*, 3rd ed. Baltimore/London: Williams and Wilkins.

Calabresi, P., and Parks, R. E., Jr. (1975). "Alkylating Agents, Antimetabolites, Hormones, and Other Antiproliferative Agents." In *The Pharmacological Basis of Therapeutics*, 5th ed., edited by L. S. Goodman and A. Gilman, 1254. New York: Macmillan Publishing Co.

Califano, Joseph A., Jr. (1979). Statement before U.S. Senate Committee on Finance, 27 March.

California Association of Hospitals and Health Systems. (1987). "Health Care Issues in California." Prepared for the California Congressional Delegation, Washington, DC, February.

California Department of Health Services. (1988). *Health Utility Management Report (HUMR), Grand Summary, July – September, 1988*. Sacramento, CA: State of California.

California Medical Association. (1976). Bureau of Research and Planning. "Physician Supply in California, December, 1975." *Socioeconomic Report* 16(8): 1.

_____. (1984). Bureau of Research and Planning. *Socioeconomic Report* 24(4): 4 (Table 2).

_____. (1987a). Bureau of Research and Planning. "Physician Supply in California, 1985." *Socioeconomic Report* 27(3): 1.

_____. (1987b). "Physician Oversupply in California: Report of the Commission on Health Manpower." In *Actions of the House of Delegates*. California Medical Association.

Clark, D. W. (1967). "Governmental Health Programs and Services." In *Preventive Medicine*, edited by D. W. Clark and B. MacMahon. Boston: Little, Brown and Company.

_____. (1981). "Health Resources: Federal Administration and Regulation." In *Preventive and Community Medicine*, 2nd ed., edited by D. W. Clark and B. MacMahon. Boston: Little, Brown and Company.

Cooper, B. S.; Worthington, N. L.; and McGee, M. F. (1976). *Compendium of National Health Expenditures Data*. DHEW Pub. No. (SSA) 76-11927. Washington, DC: U.S. Government Printing Office.

Cruz, E. P.; McDonald, G. O.; and Cole, W. H. (1956). "Prophylactic Treatment of Cancer." *Surgery* 40(2): 291 – 96.

Farber, S.; Diamond, L. K.; Mercer, R. D.; Sylvester, R. F., Jr.; and Wolff, J. A. (1948). "Temporary Remissions in Acute Leukemia in Children Produced by Folic Acid Antagonist, 4-Amino-Pteroyl-Glutamic Acid (Aminopterin)." *New England Journal of Medicine* 238(23): 787 – 93.

Friedman, E. (1986). "The Right Issues at the Wrong Time." *CHA Insight* 10(8).

Gibson, R. M., and Mueller, M. S. (1977). "National Health Expenditures, Fiscal Year 1976." *Social Security Bulletin* 40(4): 3 – 22.

Gilman, A. (1963). "The Initial Clinical Trial of Nitrogen Mustard." *American Journal of Surgery* 105(5): 574 – 78.

Gilman, A., and Philips, F. S. (1946). "The Biological Actions and Therapeutic Applications of B-Chloroethyl Amines and Sulfides." *Science* 103(2675): 409 – 15.

Goldin, A., and Carter, S. K. (1973). "Screening and Evaluation of Antitumor Agents." In *Cancer Medicine*, edited by J. F. Holland and E. Frei, 605 – 28. Philadelphia: Lea and Febiger.

Goodman, L. S., and Gilman, A. (1985). *The Pharmacological Basis of Therapeutics*. New York: Macmillan Publishing Co.

Goodman, L. S.; Wintrobe, M. M.; Damesek, W.; Goodman, M. J.; and Gilman, A. (1946). "Nitrogen Mustard Therapy. Use of Methyl-Bis (Beta Chloroethyl)amine Hydrochloride and Tris (Beta Chloroethl)amine Hydrochloride for Hodgkin's Disease, Lymphosarcoma, Leukemia, and Certain Allied and Miscellaneous Disorders." *Journal of the American Medical Association* 132(3): 126 – 32.

Haagensen, C. D. (1971). *Diseases of the Breast*, 2nd ed. Philadelphia: W. B. Saunders Company.

Holleb, A. I., and Randers-Pehrson, M. B. (1987). *Classics in Oncology*. New York: American Cancer Society.

Hunt, C. C., and Philips, F. S. (1949). "The Acute Pharmacology of Methyl-Bis(2-Chloroethyl) Amine (HN2)." *Journal of Pharmacology and Experimental Therapeutics* 95(2): 131 – 44.

Iglehart, J. K. (1984). "Health Policy Report: Cutting Costs of Health Care for the Poor of California, A Two Year Followup." *New England Journal of Medicine* 311(11): 745 – 48.

Klarman, H. E. (1967). "Financing Health and Medical Care." In *Preventive Medicine*, edited by D. W. Clark and B. MacMahon. Boston: Little, Brown and Company.

Krumbharr, E. B., and Krumbharr, H. D. (1919). "The Blood and Bone Marrow in Yellow Cross Gas (Mustard Gas) Poisoning. Changes Produced in the Bone Marrow of Fatal Cases." *Journal of Medical Research* 40(3): 497 – 508.

Marquardt, M. (1951). *Paul Ehrlich*. New York: Henry Schuman, 145 – 238.

Marshall, E. K., Jr. (1964). "Historical Perspectives in Chemotherapy." In *Advances in Chemotherapy*, edited by A. Goldin and F. Hawkings, 6 – 7. New York: Academic Press.

Melia, E. P.; Aucoin, L. M.; Duhl, L. J.; and Kurokawa, P. S. (1983). "Special Report: Competition in the Health-Care Marketplace, A Beginning in California." *New England Journal of Medicine* 308(13): 788 – 92.

Moore, G. E.; Ross, C. A.; and Stiver, R. B. (1963). "Chemotherapy as an Adjuvant to Surgery." *American Journal of Surgery* 105(5): 591 – 97.

Mrazek, R. (1970). "Adjuvant Chemotherapy with Cancer of the Breast at One Institution." In *Chemotherapy of Cancer*, edited by W. Cole, 289 – 92. Philadelphia: Lea and Febiger.

Reinhardt, U. E. (1976). "Health Manpower Policy in the United States." Paper presented at the Bicentennial Conference on Health Policy, 11 – 12 November, at the University of Pennsylvania, Philadelphia.

Roffers, M. (1986). "The Burden of Uncompensated Care." *CHA Insight* 10(17): 1.

Sudovar, S., and Sullivan, K. (1980). "National Health Insurance Issues— The Unprotected Population." In *Public Health and Community Medicine*, 3rd ed., edited by L. E. Burton, H. H. Smith, and A. W. Nichols, 549. Baltimore/London: Williams and Wilkins.

Sullivan, E. (1967). "Health Professions Educational Assistance Amendments of 1965 (P. L. 89-290)." In *Preventive Medicine*, edited by D. W. Clark and B. MacMahon, 825. Boston: Little, Brown and Company.

U.S. Department of Health and Human Services. (1986). *Directory of Facilities Obligated to Provide Uncompensated Services*, HRP-0906758. Health Resources and Services Administration. Washington, DC: U.S. Government Printing Office.

Zubrod, C. G.; Schepartz, S.; Leiter, J.; Endicott, J. M.; Carrese, L. M.; and Baker, C. G. (1966). "The Chemotherapy Program of the National Cancer Institute: History, Analysis and Plans." *Cancer Chemotherapy Reports* 50(7): 349–81.

Part II

Financing the Economic Burden of Cancer

Cancer care has a major impact on U.S. health resources. Cancer is the second leading cause of death in the United States (National Center for Health Statistics 1987). About 75 million Americans now living will eventually have cancer, which is 30 percent of the total population. Over the years, cancer will strike in approximately three out of four families (American Cancer Society 1988). A progressive increase in the number of new cases is predicted, with nearly twice as many new cases expected in the next decade (Janerich 1984). Therefore, the burden of cancer is great and it will continue into the foreseeable future.

The economic burden of cancer and the means for financing that burden are the subjects of Part II. Chapter 3 was written by Dorothy P. Rice, Thomas A. Hodgson, and Frank Capell, who are well known for their work on the costs of illness. They examine the economic and social burden of cancer. By employing the prevalence-based approach, the authors estimate the economic costs of cancer, including direct and indirect costs, at $72.5 billion, comprising 10.7 percent of the economic costs of all illnesses in the United States in 1985. In addition to total costs, Rice, Hodgson, and Capell calculate, for the first time, the burden of cancer in California, the most populous state in the United States.

One attempt to address the economic burden of illness has

been the initiation of cost-containment measures. The prospective payment system, introduced in 1983, represents a major policy change for the Medicare program. It was designed to encourage more cost-effective care without compromising the quality of care. The impact of PPS—especially the impact on cancer care, which represents a major Medicare expenditure—is a major concern today. Chapter 4 was written by Stephen F. Jencks, who is Acting Director, Office of Research, for the Health Care and Financing Administration, the agency that administers Medicare. He discusses the impact of PPS and diagnosis-related groups on cancer care, prevention, and research. He concludes that there are many difficult financing issues to be resolved, including DRG payment weights, outlier reimbursement, and adjustments for severity of illness.

Lester Breslow, the author of Chapter 5, is a well-known researcher in cancer and health issues. He echoes Jencks by stating that clarifying and resolving key reimbursement issues will be highly important in meeting our objectives in cancer control. Breslow focuses on cancer prevention, screening, and treatment and describes how the present patterns of reimbursement impede progress in cancer control. He discusses four reimbursement issues—incorporation of preventive services into reimbursement mechanisms, pricing for preventive services, state-of-the-art diagnosis and treatment, and commercialization—in his argument that prevention is the key to making progress in our fight against cancer.

REFERENCES

American Cancer Society. (1988). *Cancer Facts and Figures—1988*. New York: American Cancer Society.

Janerich, D. T. (1984). "Forecasting Cancer Trends to Optimize Control Strategies." *Journal of the National Cancer Institute* 72(6): 1317–21.

National Center for Health Statistics. (1987). "Advance Report of Final Mortality Statistics, 1985," *Monthly Vital Statistics Report* 36, no. 5 (Suppl.). DHHS Pub. No. (PHS) 87-1120. Washington, DC: U.S. Government Printing Office.

3 The Economic Burden of Cancer, 1985: United States and California

Dorothy P. Rice, Thomas A. Hodgson, and Frank Capell

ABSTRACT.   Cancer is the second leading cause of death in the United States and in California, and the economic burden is great. Employing the prevalence-based approach, the total economic costs of cancer, including direct and indirect costs, are estimated at $72.5 billion, comprising 10.7 percent of the economic costs of all illnesses in the United States in 1985. Of the $72.5 billion, direct costs, including hospital and nursing home care, physicians and other professional services, and drugs, comprised 25 percent of the total; morbidity costs, 10 percent; and mortality costs, 65 percent. For California, the total economic costs of cancer amounted to $7.3 billion. The distribution by type of costs in California is similar to that for the United States.

The burden of illness and disease in general, and of cancer in particular, is great. From the individual's point of view, the burden includes pain and suffering, reduced quality of life, and high monetary payments for medical care, as well as losses associated with reduction in ability to work or keep house, and premature mortality. The individual's family and friends also suffer emotional trauma, grief, and financial losses.

From society's point of view, it must bear the negative social consequences of suffering of the patients, families, and friends, as well as the costs of resources used for medical care and the losses due to morbidity, disability, and premature mortality. The social and economic implications of disease include pain and suffering, illness and disability, resources devoted to prevention, research, detection, diagnosis, and treatment, premature death and years of life lost, and billions of dollars of economic output forgone annually because of lost human resources.

This chapter focuses on malignant neoplasms—cancer—its staggering costs to society and its relationship to the economic costs of all illness in the United States and in California in 1985.

BACKGROUND

Cancer is a large group of diseases that are characterized by uncontrolled growth and the spread of abnormal cells affecting many different body systems. There are more than 5 million Americans alive today who have a history of cancer. Of this total, 3 million were diagnosed five or more years ago, most of whom can be considered cured. About 965,000 people were diagnosed as having cancer in 1987 and about 49 percent were expected to be alive five years after diagnosis and treatment. By contrast, only 20 percent were alive five years after treatment in the 1930s (American Cancer Society 1987).

Significant improvements have been made in survival rates for some cancers: acute lymphocytic leukemia in children, Hodgkin's disease, Burkett's lymphoma, Ewing's sarcoma (a form of bone cancer), Wilms' tumor (a kidney cancer in children), rhabdomyosarcoma (a cancer in certain muscle tissue), choricarcinoma (placental cancer), testicular cancer, ovarian cancer, and osteogenic sarcoma. Despite this progress, there has been a steady rise in the age-adjusted national death rate for malignant neoplasms from 157 per 100,000 population in 1950 to 171 in 1985 (National Cancer Institute 1988). The major reason for this increase is the continued rise in deaths due to lung cancer, accounting for 27.6 percent of the deaths from all cancers in 1985 (National Center for Health Statistics 1987). Age-adjusted cancer death rates for other major sites are leveling off and declining in some cases.

Cancer has been and currently is the second leading cause of death in the United States and in California, following diseases of the heart. In 1985, 461,563 persons died from cancer, accounting for 22 percent of the 2.1 million deaths in the country (National

Table 3.1: Cancer Deaths: Number, Percent of Total Deaths, and
Rank as Leading Cause of Death by Age, United States, 1985

Age Group	Number	Percent of Total	Rank Order in Age Group
United States, Total	461,563[a]	22.2%	2
1–4	543	7.4	3
5–14	1,183	13.2	2
15–24	2,142	5.6	4
25–44	20,026	17.0	2
45–64	138,829	34.4	1
65 and over	298,683	20.3	2

Source: National Center for Health Statistics, "Advance Report of Final
Mortality Statistics, 1985," *Monthly Vital Statistics Report* 36, no. 5 (Suppl.),
DHHS Pub. No. (PHS) 87-1120 (Washington, DC: U.S. Government Printing
Office, 1987).
[a]Includes 114 deaths under one year of age and 43 deaths with age not stated.

Center for Health Statistics 1987). Cancer's rank as a leading
cause of death in the United States varies by age group. For the
population aged 45 – 64 years, cancer was the leading cause of
death; it accounted for 34 percent of the deaths in that age group.
For persons aged 15 – 24 years, it ranked fourth, causing 6 percent
of total deaths in that age group. The ranking of cancer deaths in
1985 and proportion of total deaths in each age group is shown in
Table 3.1.

In addition to incidence, prevalence, survival rates, and
deaths, the burden of cancer can be measured in economic terms.
The economic costs of cancer are expressed as follows:

- Direct costs—amounts spent for medical care in the prevention, diagnosis, and treatment of cancer patients
- Indirect costs—the value of output lost or forgone due to
  illness, disability (morbidity costs), and premature death
  (mortality costs)
- Psychosocial costs—intangible effects, such as pain and
  suffering and deterioration in the quality of life, which are
  not reflected in the direct and indirect costs. These psychosocial costs are difficult, if not impossible, to quantify.

The economic costs of cancer have been estimated in the past
as a major diagnostic category of the total economic costs of illness
for 1963, 1972, 1975, and 1980 (Rice 1966; Cooper and Rice 1976;

Paringer and Berk 1977; Rice, Hodgson, and Kopstein 1985). Estimates of the costs of cancer by cancer site have also been made in the past for 1977 and 1980 (Rice and Hodgson 1981; Hodgson 1984).

This chapter updates to 1985 the authors' previous estimates of the economic costs of malignant neoplasms, and, for the first time, comparable cost estimates are made for the state of California. National data on the economic costs of neoplasms (malignant and benign) for 1985 were published by the National Cancer Institute (NCI) in its *1986 Annual Cancer Statistics Review* (National Cancer Institute 1987). The national data presented here were estimated in more detail and therefore vary slightly from the NCI published figures. The costs of benign neoplasms are excluded from this study.

The costs of neoplasms presented here are prevalence-based costs; they provide an estimate of the direct and indirect economic burden incurred in 1985 as a result of the prevalence of disease during the same period. The methodology closely follows that developed originally by Rice (1966) to allocate expenditures among diagnoses, but it has been amended to include additional sources of data. The methodology is briefly described in the Appendix at the end of this chapter.

FINDINGS

Direct Medical Care Costs

In 1985, direct medical care cancer costs amounted to $18.1 billion and comprised almost 5 percent of the total personal health spending in the United States (Table 3.2 and Figure 3.1). Hospital care of cancer patients accounted for $12.1 billion, or two-thirds of this total. In contrast, hospital care spending for all illnesses comprised 45 percent of total medical spending in the United States. This relative difference is due to the higher rate of hospitalization and longer stays for cancer patients compared with many other illnesses. Physicians' services for cancer patients amounted to $4.1 billion (23 percent of the total) and considerably lesser amounts were spent for nursing home care ($919 million), drugs ($656 million), and other professional services ($326 million).

Medical care cancer costs in California amounted to $2.2 billion in 1985 and almost 5 percent of total spending for medical

Table 3.2: Total Medical Care and Cancer Expenditures by Type of Expenditure: United States and California, 1985

| | United States | | | | California | | | |
| | Total Medical Care | | Cancer | | Total Medical Care | | Cancer | |
Type of Expenditure	Amount (millions)	Percent Distribution	Amount (millions)	Percent Distribution	Amount (millions)	Percent Distribution	Amount (millions)	Percent Distribution
Total	$371,400	100.0%	$18,104	100.0%	$46,620	100.0%	$2,176	100.0%
Hospital care	166,700	44.9	12,118	66.9	19,087	40.9	1,388	63.8
Physicians' services	82,800	22.3	4,082	22.5	12,487	26.8	616	28.3
Nursing home care	35,200	9.5	919	5.1	2,975	6.4	78	3.6
Drugs	28,500	7.7	659	3.6	3,348	7.2	77	3.5
Other professional services	39,700	10.7	326	1.8	2,101	4.5	17	0.8
Other health services	18,500	5.0	—	—	6,622	14.2	—	—

Note: Numbers may not add to totals due to rounding.

Figure 3.1: Medical Care Expenditures, All Illnesses and Cancer, United States, 1985

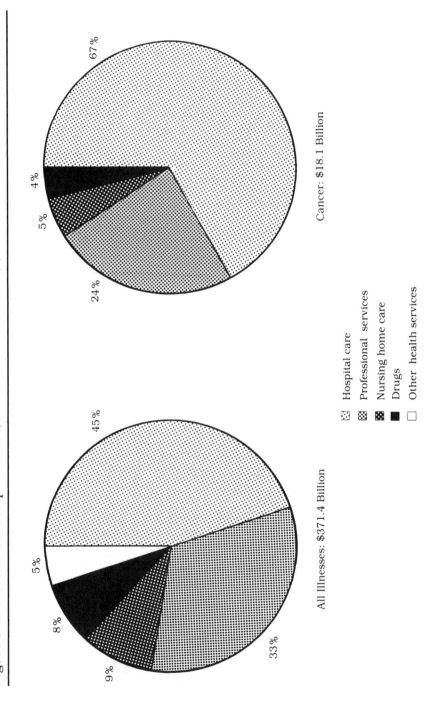

All Illnesses: $371.4 Billion

Cancer: $18.1 Billion

Hospital care

Professional services

Nursing home care

Drugs

Other health services

care (Table 3.2). The distribution of these costs in California by type of expenditures shows relatively smaller proportions are spent for hospital and nursing home care than for the nation as a whole. For physicians' services, however, the proportion is higher in California.

Morbidity Costs

As one component of indirect costs, morbidity costs represent the value of losses in output for people who are ill and disabled and unable to work. We used average earnings by age and sex and ascribed a value to housekeeping services for those who are unable to keep house because of illness and disability. Morbidity and disability from cancer in the United States in 1985 resulted in $7.2 billion of lost output, representing 8.9 percent of the morbidity costs for all diseases (Table 3.3). For California, cancer morbidity costs amounted to $875 million, comprising 9.8 percent of morbidity costs for all diseases. As indicated earlier, cancer direct costs represent almost 5 percent of the total medical care expenditures for all diseases in the United States and in California. Although we are spending more for cancer than for many other diseases, cancer results in relatively more illness, disability, and lost productivity than most other illnesses.

Mortality Costs

A second component of indirect costs, mortality costs, represents the value of losses to productivity for people who die prematurely. If an individual had not died, he or she would have continued to be productive for a number of years depending on age of death. It is the present value of these future losses that constitutes the mortality costs.

For mortality, the estimated cost or value of productivity lost to society is the product of the number of deaths and the expected value of an individual's future earnings, with sex and age at death taken into account. This method of derivation must consider for each death a variety of variables: life expectancy, labor force participation rates, earnings, imputed values for housekeeping services, and an appropriate discount rate to convert lifetime earnings to present worth. (A brief description of the methodology is included in the appendix at the end of this chapter.)

In 1985, 461,563 persons died from cancer in the United States, representing a loss of 7.2 million years (Table 3.4). The

Table 3.3: Economic Costs of All Illnesses and Cancer, by Type
of Cost: United States and California, 1985

	All Illnesses		Cancer		
Type of Cost	Amounts (millions)	Percent Distribution	Amount (millions)	Percent Distribution	Percent of All Illnesses
United States					
Total	$679,712	100.0%	$72,494	100.0%	10.7
Direct	371,400	54.6	18,104	25.0	4.9
Indirect	308,312	45.4	54,390	75.0	17.6
Morbidity	80,850	11.9	7,170	9.9	8.9
Mortality[a]	227,462	33.5	47,220	65.1	20.8
California					
Total	78,671	100.0	7,257	100.0	9.2
Direct	46,620	59.3	2,176	30.0	4.7
Indirect	32,051	40.7	5,081	70.0	15.9
Morbidity	8,920	11.3	875	12.0	9.8
Mortality[a]	23,131	29.4	4,206	58.0	18.2

[a]Discounted at 4 percent.

number of deaths increased sharply with age and was higher for
males for each age group shown, except among persons 25 to 44
years of age. Males accounted for 53 percent of the deaths from
cancer, and 65 percent of the deaths occurred at 65 years of age
and over. Cancer deaths represented 22 percent of all deaths, but
the proportion varied with age. Only 4 percent of the deaths under
age 25 were due to cancer, compared with 17 percent for the
25 – 44 age group, 34 percent of the 45 – 64 age group, and 20
percent of the deaths in the 65 years and older age group.

Applying expected lifetime earnings by age and gender to the
461,563 cancer deaths in the United States in 1985 results in a
loss of $47 billion to the economy at a 4 percent discount rate (the
rate by which the present value of future earnings can be estimated). Costs per cancer death amounted to $102,305. For the
246,914 males who died from cancer in 1985, an estimated total of
3.5 million person-years were lost, valued at $26 billion. About
214,650 females died, representing a loss of 3.7 million person-
years, or 52 percent of all the years lost. Because of the higher
earnings of males, however, losses for females are somewhat
lower, amounting to $21 billion. Thus, males account for 53 per-
cent of the deaths, 48 percent of the person-years lost, and 55

Table 3.4: Deaths, Person-Years Lost, and Mortality Costs by Age and Sex: All Causes and Cancer, United States, 1985

Age and Sex	All Causes of Death			Cancer		
	Number of Deaths	Person-Years Lost (thousands)	Mortality Costs[b] (millions)	Number of Deaths	Person-Years Lost (thousands)	Mortality Costs[b] (millions)
Total	2,086,440[a]	33,253	$227,462	461,563[a]	7,210	$47,220
Under 25	94,237	6,149	49,172	3,982	244	2,295
25–44	117,667	4,772	70,758	20,026	799	10,684
45–64	403,114	8,843	82,197	138,829	3,084	27,296
65 and over	1,470,545	13,490	25,334	298,683	3,082	6,946
Males	1,097,758[a]	18,044	154,231	246,914[a]	3,467	25,953
Under 25	60,846	3,756	35,092	2,333	136	1,476
25–44	80,848	3,150	53,693	9,344	346	5,939
45–64	251,031	5,067	54,697	74,883	1,486	15,570
65 and over	704,542	6,071	10,749	160,333	1,499	2,969
Females	988,682[a]	15,209	73,231	214,649[a]	3,743	21,267
Under 25	33,391	2,392	14,080	1,649	108	819
25–44	36,819	1,623	17,065	10,682	454	4,745
45–64	152,083	3,776	27,501	63,946	1,598	11,726
65 and over	766,003	7,419	14,586	138,350	1,584	3,977

Source: 1985 deaths from the National Center for Health Statistics.

Note: Numbers may not add to totals due to rounding.

[a]Includes the following deaths with age not noted: All deaths—877 total. 491 males and 386 females; cancer deaths—43 total. 21 males and 22 females.

[b]Discounted at 4 percent.

percent of the productivity losses. Premature deaths due to cancer are very costly to the nation.

The number of cancer deaths, person-years lost, and discounted earnings vary by age: the highest number and proportion of deaths are among the aged, representing almost two-thirds of the total (Figure 3.2). The total person-years lost, a function of both age and number of deaths, shows a different picture. Persons 65 years of age or over who died would have had relatively few remaining years of life; their deaths represented 43 percent of the person-years lost. In terms of lost earnings, however, this age group accounts for only 15 percent of the total. On the other hand, costs for the 158,855 persons aged 25 to 64 (the highest productive years) represented 80 percent of the total, and costs per cancer death amounted to $239,086. The much higher earnings losses for those who died from cancer under age 65 are the result of their considerably higher expected lifetime earnings remaining at the time of death.

Deaths from all causes and from cancer, person-years lost, and mortality costs for California are listed in Table 3.5. A total of 45,609 deaths in 1985 were due to cancer, resulting in 733,000 person-years lost, and $4.2 billion in productivity losses. Cancer deaths comprised 23 percent of the total deaths in California. Slightly more than half of the total cancer deaths (52 percent) were males, accounting for less than half (47 percent) of the person-years lost, and 57 percent of the mortality costs. The higher costs for men are mainly due to their higher earnings.

The distributions of cancer deaths in California, person-years lost, and costs for selected cancer sites are listed in Table 3.6 and compared in Figure 3.3. Deaths from lung cancer and cancer of other respiratory and intrathoracic organs took the largest toll: 12,497 deaths, 193,000 person-years lost, and $1 billion in lost productivity. Cancer of the digestive organs and peritoneum resulted in 11,412 deaths in 1985 and accounted for 161,000 person-years lost, and over $800 million in lost productivity.

The leading cause of cancer deaths among males in 1985 in California was cancer of the respiratory and intrathoracic organs (33 percent), followed by cancer of the digestive organs and peritoneum (26 percent). The reverse was the case for women: cancer of the digestive organs comprised 24 percent of total cancer deaths, and cancer of the respiratory and intrathoracic organs comprised 21 percent, followed closely by cancer of the breast (18.5 percent).

Figure 3.2: Cancer Mortality Losses by Age, United States, 1985

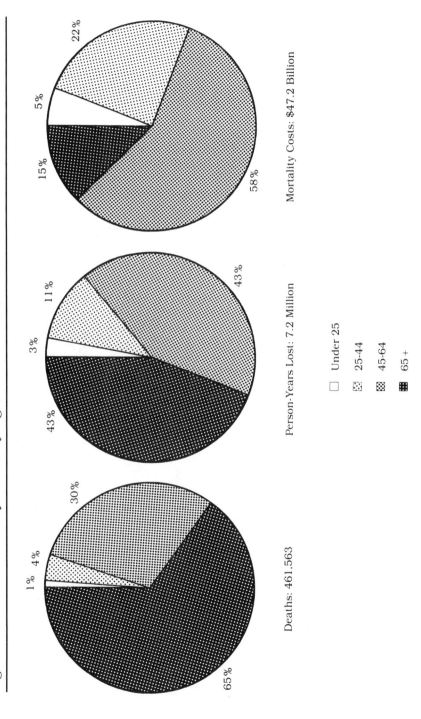

Deaths: 461.563

Person-Years Lost: 7.2 Million

Mortality Costs: $47.2 Billion

☐ Under 25

⬚ 25-44

▨ 45-64

▦ 65 +

Table 3.5: Deaths, Person-Years Lost, and Mortality Costs by Age and Sex: All Causes and Cancer, California, 1985

Age and Sex	All Causes of Death			Cancer		
	Number of Deaths	Person-Years Lost (thousands)	Mortality Costs[b] (millions)	Number of Deaths	Person-Years Lost (thousands)	Mortality Costs[b] (millions)
Total	201,815[a]	3,456	$23,131	45,609	733	$4,206
Under 25	10,759	698	6,211	472	29	289
25–44	14,377	586	8,428	2,305	92	1,180
45–64	38,725	855	6,780	13,762	308	2,259
65 and over	137,796	1,317	1,712	29,070	304	478
Males	106,368[a]	1,887	16,397	23,755	343	2,379
Under 25	7,031	431	4,427	283	17	187
25–44	10,181	401	6,601	1,123	42	694
45–64	23,823	484	4,626	7,124	142	1,291
65 and over	65,214	571	743	15,225	142	207
Females	95,447[a]	1,569	6,734	21,854	390	1,827
Under 25	3,728	267	1,784	189	12	102
25–44	4,196	185	1,827	1,182	50	486
45–64	14,902	371	2,154	6,638	166	968
65 and over	72,582	746	969	13,845	162	271

Source: 1985 deaths from Vital Statistics of California, 1985. Department of Health and Human Services. Health and Welfare Agency. State of California. September 1987.
[a]Includes 158 deaths with age not stated, 119 males and 39 females.
[b]Discounted at 4 percent.

Table 3.6: Cancer Deaths, Person-Years Lost, and Costs by Site: California, 1985

Site	ICD Code	Deaths			Person-Years Lost (thousands)			Mortality Costs[b] (millions)		
		Total	Males	Females	Total	Males	Females	Total	Males	Females
Total		45,609	23,755	21,854	733	343	390	$4,206	$2,379	$1,827
Lips, oral cavity, and pharynx	140–149	873	502	371	15	8	7	92	62	30
Digestive organs and peritoneum	150–159	11,412	6,058	5,354	161	82	79	806	518	288
Respiratory and intrathoracic organs	160–165	12,497	7,950	4,547	193	111	82	1,024	671	353
Breast	174–175	4,068	25	4,043	81	a	81	441	2	439
Genital organs	179–187	4,863	2,578	2,285	69	26	43	316	99	217
Urinary organs	188–189	1,697	1,101	596	22	14	8	109	77	32
All other and unspecified sites	170–173 190–199	5,810	3,145	2,665	111	59	52	832	557	275
Lymphatic and hematopoietic tissue	200–208	4,389	2,396	1,993	81	43	38	586	393	193

Source: 1985 deaths from *Vital Statistics of California, 1985.* Department of Health and Human Services. Health and Welfare Agency. State of California. September 1987.
Note: Numbers may not add to totals due to rounding.
[a]Less than 500.
[b]Discounted at 4 percent.

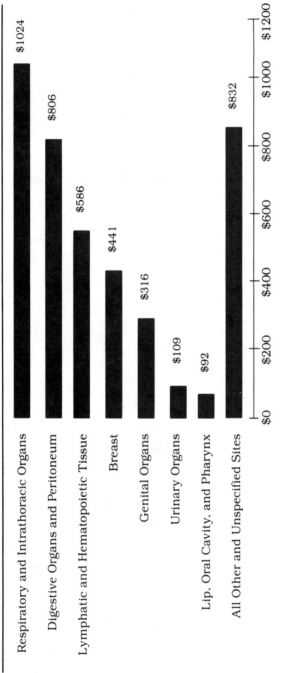

Figure 3.3: Cancer Mortality Losses, California, 1985

Respiratory and Intrathoracic Organs — $1024

Digestive Organs and Peritoneum — $806

Lymphatic and Hematopoietic Tissue — $586

Breast — $441

Genital Organs — $316

Urinary Organs — $109

Lip, Oral Cavity, and Pharynx — $92

All Other and Unspecified Sites — $832

Amount in Millions of Dollars

$0 $200 $400 $600 $800 $1000 $1200

Total Indirect Costs

The total indirect costs of cancer, morbidity and mortality costs combined, amounted to $54.4 billion in the United States and $5.1 billion in California in 1985 (Table 3.3). These amounts are considerably higher than the direct costs of cancer. For all illnesses in the United States and in California, direct costs are higher than indirect costs. This differential reflects cancer's high rate of premature mortality compared with other diseases.

Total Economic Costs

Total economic costs of cancer, including direct and indirect costs, are estimated at $72.5 billion, comprising 10.7 percent of the economic costs of all illnesses in the United States in 1985 (Figure 3.4). Of the $72.5 billion, direct costs comprised 25 percent of the total; morbidity costs, 10 percent; and mortality costs, 65 percent.

As noted earlier, cancer is characterized by a higher premature mortality rate than many other diseases, resulting in significantly higher indirect costs relative to medical care expenditures. In 1985, the total economic costs of illness amounted to $680 billion, of which direct costs comprised 55 percent of the total and indirect costs comprised 45 percent.

For California, the total economic costs of cancer amounted to $7.3 billion, or 9.2 percent of the total economic costs of all illnesses. Costs in California are distributed as follows: direct costs, 30 percent; morbidity costs, 12 percent; and mortality costs, 58 percent.

COST IMPLICATIONS

Large figures representing billions of dollars have limited meaning for most people. To put into perspective the $18.1 billion spent on direct medical care for cancer in 1985, Table 3.7 presents personal consumption expenditures for selected items in the United States during the same year (U.S. Department of Commerce 1986). The table shows, for example, that the cost of cancer care was 15 percent of the amount spent for household utilities, one-fifth of spending for gasoline and oil, almost three-fifths of expenditures on tobacco, and almost two-thirds of spending for legal services. On the other hand, spending for cancer care was 17 percent higher than the amount the nation's consumers spent on higher educa-

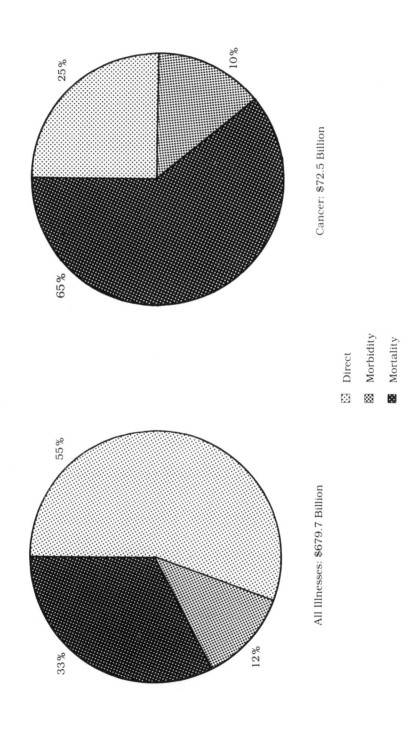

Figure 3.4: Economic Costs of All Illnesses and Cancer, United States, 1985

All Illnesses: $679.7 Billion

Cancer: $72.5 Billion

Direct

Morbidity

Mortality

Table 3.7: Personal Consumption Expenditures for Selected
Items, United States, 1985

Item	Amount (billions)	Per Capita Expenditures	Ratio of Cancer Expenditures to Expenditures for Item
Household utilities[a]	$121.2	$508	0.15
Furniture and household equipment[b]	105.6	442	0.17
Gasoline and oil	91.9	385	0.20
Alcoholic beverages	55.5	232	0.33
Tobacco products	31.8	133	0.57
Legal services	28.1	118	0.64
Cancer medical care	18.1	76	1.00
Higher education	15.5	65	1.17
Magazines, newspapers, and sheet music	13.2	55	1.37
Bank service charges[c]	11.7	49	1.55
Admissions to spectator amusements	9.7	41	1.87

Source: U.S. Department of Commerce, *Survey of Current Business* 66, no. 7 (July 1986): Table 2.4.

[a]Includes electricity, gas, water and sanitary services, and fuel oil and coal.

[b]Includes furniture; kitchen and other household appliances; china, glassware, tableware, and utensils; and other durable and semidurable furnishings.

[c]Includes bank service charges, trust services, and safe deposit box rental.

tion, 37 percent more than the amount spent on magazines and newspapers, and 87 percent more than the amount spent for admissions to a variety of spectator amusements.

To put in perspective the aggregate amount of indirect costs of cancer, the costs are compared in Table 3.8 to wages and salaries in selected industries in the United States in 1985. The value of productive labor lost to morbidity and mortality from cancer was $47.1 billion. This is a significant diminution in the nation's capacity to produce goods and services. By comparison, the labor lost to cancer is sufficient to provide almost half the needs of the construction industry and more than twice the labor required by real estate, legal, and educational services. Even a relatively small reduction in indirect costs of cancer would increase the value of productive labor by several billion dollars and the capacity of the economy to supply additional goods and services. It is clear that the indirect costs of cancer are large and represent a significant

Table 3.8: Wages and Salaries by Industry, 1985

Industry	Amount (billions)	Ratio of Amount for Cancer to Amount for Item
Construction	$102.1	0.46
Transportation[a]	72.5	0.65
Cancer morbidity and mortality	47.1	1.00
Food and kindred products manufacturing	33.5	1.41
Telephone and telegraph	32.0	1.47
Motor vehicles and equipment	29.3	1.61
Textile mill, apparel and other textile manufacturing	25.1	1.88
Real estate	21.6	2.18
Legal services	21.5	2.19
Educational services	19.9	2.37

Source: U.S. Department of Commerce, *Survey of Current Business* 66, no. 7 (July 1986): Table 6.5B.

[a]Includes railroad, local and interurban passenger transit, trucking and warehousing, water, air, pipelines (except natural gas), and other transportation services.

loss of resources and diminution of the nation's capacity in terms of production of goods and services.

Over the years, cancer costs have increased relative to those of most other diseases. They accounted for 1 percent of the total costs of all diseases in 1900 (Berk and Paringer 1977a), 4 percent in 1930 (Berk and Paringer 1977b), 9 percent in 1975 (Paringer and Berk 1977), and 11 percent in 1985 (Table 3.3). In 1900, cancer was the tenth leading cause of death and accounted for less than 3 percent of all deaths. In 1930, cancer accounted for 9 percent of all deaths and was the sixth leading cause of death. By 1975 and 1985, cancer was the second leading cause of death, exceeded only by deaths from diseases of the circulatory system. In 1975, cancer accounted for 19 percent of all deaths; in 1985, the proportion of total deaths was 22 percent.

Future levels of cancer costs depend on a variety of factors including incidence, mortality, and survival rates; utilization and cost of medical care; new cancer therapies and technologies; the size and age distribution of the population; environmental and behavioral factors; and scientific breakthroughs in prevention and treatment.

Economic costs are potential benefits of reduced cancer morbidity and mortality. Direct costs represent resources that could be allocated to other uses, and indirect costs are the value of idle resources and output. Knowledge of the costs of cancer and of specific diseases is an aid to more rational decision making with respect to allocating scarce resources among competing programs.

APPENDIX: METHODOLOGY

Details concerning the methodology for calculating the economic costs of illness may be found in the authors' previous articles on this subject (Rice 1966; Cooper and Rice 1976; Rice and Hodgson 1981; Hodgson and Meiners 1982; Hodgson 1983; Rice, Hodgson, and Kopstein 1985). This appendix provides a brief description of the methodology and data sources used to estimate the economic costs of cancer that were presented in this chapter.

Direct Costs

National health expenditures, by type of expenditure, are published annually by the Health Care Financing Administration (1987). Total expenditures in 1985 for hospital care, physicians' services, and the other direct costs of illness are distributed by diagnosis (cancer) according to utilization and costs, using consistent data sources for each type of expenditure. Expenditures in community hospitals, for example, were allocated to cancer in proportion to the number of days of care attributable to cancer from the National Hospital Discharge Survey multiplied by the expense per patient day. Utilization of other medical care services, weighted by unit costs, determined the share of total direct medical expenditures assigned to cancer.

Direct costs of cancer for California are based on the state expenditures for medical care by type of expenditures for 1982 published by the Health Care Financing Administration (Levit 1985). To estimate 1985 levels, the 1982 expenditures were inflated according to the increase by type in national health expenditures. The direct costs of cancer in California are based on the proportion of national expenditures by type allocated to cancer.

Morbidity Costs

Morbidity losses are estimated separately for those who are currently employed, housekeepers, persons unable to work because of ill health, and the institutionalized population. Among the currently employed, days lost from work due to cancer are converted to years lost by age and sex and multiplied by age- and gender-specific estimates of average annual earnings to obtain lost earnings for this group. Days of bed disability (confinement to bed) suffered by those who have cancer who usually keep house are also converted to years, and then multiplied by age-specific values of housekeepers' services, to obtain morbidity costs for this group. The number of persons unable to work (by age and sex) is multiplied by employment rates and average annual earnings and by housekeeping rates and housekeeping values to determine indirect morbidity costs among members of this group. A similar procedure is applied to the institutionalized population to estimate morbidity costs by institution. These separate components of morbidity costs are aggregated to obtain a total cancer morbidity cost figure.

Cancer morbidity costs for California were based on the share of total national morbidity costs allocated to cancer, adjusted for the differential in wages and salaries for Californians compared with that for the nation.

Mortality Costs

To obtain the indirect costs of mortality, the numbers of deaths in 1985 (by age and sex) are multiplied by the present value of lifetime earnings (also by age and sex). The number of person-years lost due to premature mortality is the product of the number of deaths and life expectancy at the midyear of the age group. This method accounts for life expectancy, labor force participation and housekeeping rates, earnings, imputed values of housekeeping services, and discount rates for each age group and gender. Estimates for 1985 include imputed housekeeping values for women and men in the labor force who have household responsibilities.

The number of cancer deaths by age and sex in the United States in 1985 were obtained from the National Center for Health Statistics (1987). The 1985 California deaths by cancer site were provided by the California Department of Health Services (1987).

REFERENCES

American Cancer Society. (1987). *Cancer Facts and Figures—1987*. New York: American Cancer Society.

Berk, A., and Paringer, L. (1977a). "Costs of Illness and Disease, 1900." Report No. B5. Washington, DC: Public Services Laboratory, George Washington University.

_____. (1976b). "Costs of Illness and Disease; Fiscal Year 1930." Report No. 4. Washington, DC: Public Service Laboratory, George Washington University.

California Department of Health Services. (1987). "Vital Statistics of California, 1985." Sacramento, CA: Health and Welfare Agency.

Cooper, B. S., and Rice, D. P. (1976). "The Economic Cost of Illness Revisited." *Social Security Bulletin* 39(2):21 – 36.

Health Care Financing Administration. (1987). "National Health Expenditures, 1986 – 2000." *Health Care Financing Review* 8(4):1 – 36.

Hodgson, T. A. (1983). "The State of the Art of Cost-of-Illness Estimates." *Advances in Health Economics and Health Services* 4:129 – 64.

_____. (1984). "The Economic Burden of Cancer." In *Proceedings of the American Cancer Society Fourth National Conference on Human Values & Cancer*. New York: American Cancer Society.

Hodgson, T. A., and Meiners, M. (1982). "Cost-of-Illness Methodology: A Guide to Current Practices and Procedures." *Milbank Memorial Fund Quarterly* 60(3):429 – 62.

Levit, K. R. (1985). "Personal Health Care Expenditures by State: 1966 – 82." *Health Care Financing Review* 6(4):1 – 48.

National Cancer Institute. (1987). *1986 Annual Cancer Statistics Review*. National Institutes of Health. NIH Pub. No. 87-2789. Washington, DC: U.S. Government Printing Office.

_____. (1988). *1987 Annual Cancer Statistics Review*. National Institutes of Health. NIH Pub. No. 88-2789. Washington, DC: U.S. Government Printing Office.

National Center for Health Statistics (1987). "Advance Report of Final Mortality Statistics, 1985." *Monthly Vital Statistics Report* 36, no. 5 (Suppl.). DHHS Pub. No. (PHS) 87-1120. Washington, DC: U.S. Government Printing Office.

Paringer, L., and Berk, A. (1977). "Cost of Illness and Disease, Fiscal Year 1975." Report No. 2. Washington, DC: Public Services Laboratory, Georgetown University.

Rice, D. P. (1966). "Estimating the Cost of Illness." Health Economics Series No. 6. PHS Pub. No. 947-6. Washington, DC: U.S. Government Printing Office.

Rice, D. P., and Hodgson, T. A. (1981). "Social and Economic Implications of Cancer in the United States." National Center for Health Statistics. *Vital and Health Statistics*, Series 3, No. 20. DHHS Pub. No. (PHS) 81-1404. Washington, DC: U.S. Government Printing Office.

Rice, D. P.; Hodgson, T. A.; and Kopstein, A. N. (1985). "The Economic Costs of Illness: A Replication and Update." *Health Care Financing Review* 7(1):61 – 80.

U.S. Department of Commerce. (1986). *Survey of Current Business* 66 (7): Tables 2, 4, and 6.5B.

4 Prospective Payment and Cancer

Stephen F. Jencks

ABSTRACT.   The Medicare prospective payment system and its use of DRGs to determine payments for hospital care has revolutionized provider awareness of cost-effectiveness in medical care. This chapter is intended to help those interested in cancer research, prevention, and care to understand this revolution. The author discusses the nature of PPS and DRGs. Three major issues in PPS are considered: severity of illness, purpose of care, and intensity of care. Finally, issues of special pertinence to cancer are discussed, including protocol patients, excluded facilities, capitation, prevention, and quality of care.

The Medicare prospective payment system and its use of diagnosis-related groups to determine payments for hospital care has revolutionized provider awareness of cost-effectiveness in medical care; and revolutions are rarely either smooth or painless. The purpose of this chapter is to help those interested in cancer research, prevention, and care to understand this revolution. Increased understanding should help to reduce unnecessary anxiety and contribute to constructive proposals for change.

THE NATURE OF PPS AND DRGs

Goals of the Payment Policy

Understanding the impact of PPS requires an understanding of the

---

The views herein are the author's and should not be represented as those of the Health Care Financing Administration.

goals of Medicare payment policy (Jencks et al. 1984). Payment policy should accomplish the following goals:

1. Control overall expenditures, particularly through providing incentives for efficiency.

2. Be fair to patients by paying enough to provide access to quality care and by avoiding any possible incentive for providers to discriminate against patients with particular diseases or personal characteristics.

3. Be fair to hospitals by paying enough to provide quality care in reasonably efficient facilities.

4. Provide incentives for providing quality care. (This goal has only recently achieved prominence, and ways to attain it are still unclear.)

The Nature of Prospective Payment

The prospective payment system was designed primarily to provide incentives for efficiency while maintaining fairness to patients and hospitals. In the past, Medicare determined the payment for inpatient care after the care was rendered, and then paid its best estimate of the actual cost of treatment (cost-based reimbursement). Under PPS, Medicare fixes the amount that it will pay for the care of a patient with particular characteristics at the beginning of the year (prospectively). The incentive for efficiency is clear: the hospital profits by not delivering services. But the risk is equally clear: that hospitals will profit not only by reducing unnecessary services but also by skimping on services that the patient needs. This concern has generated unprecedented attention to quality of care issues. Indeed, the future may record that the most important consequence of cost containment in general, and PPS in particular, was an increased public interest in measuring the effectiveness of care.

Diagnosis-related groups are a key part of PPS. DRGs form a classification system with about 475 mutually exclusive categories (the number changes yearly) into which all hospital discharges can be classified. The DRG system was created with a principal goal of making categories as homogeneous as possible with regard to resource consumption, and the PPS payment for a hospitalization is based on the DRG to which the discharge is assigned.

A computer program, called a Grouper, actually assigns a discharge to a DRG using a classification algorithm that is based primarily on discharge diagnoses (both the principal diagnosis and certain additional diagnoses) and the procedures performed. Sometimes other factors define a DRG, such as whether the patient was alive on discharge or whether the patient was under 17 years old. Some DRGs are very precisely defined (e.g., cholecystectomy without common duct exploration is distinguished from cholecystectomy with common duct exploration), while other DRGs are fairly broad (all strokes, for example, are grouped together). Some DRGs are defined by a principal diagnosis of cancer (e.g., lung cancer); others are largely composed of patients with cancer but include some other conditions as well (e.g., large bowel surgery); still others may contain patients with cancers but are defined by conditions that have no particular relationship to cancer (e.g., diabetes). Cancer stage is generally not available in the diagnostic data although diagnosis data often contain some related information.

Before PPS, hospitals had rather limited incentives to record diagnoses accurately. Now, recording certain diagnoses can place a patient in a DRG with higher payments, and the order in which diagnoses are recorded also influences the DRG assignment. Thus, DRG-based payments have created strong incentives to record all diagnoses that are present and even some that are not, as well as to manipulate the order in which diagnoses are reported. This kind of manipulation is known as "DRG creep," and there is intense controversy as to its magnitude and meaning. Some research suggests that much of what critics have called creep is actually more accurate coding (Lloyd and Rissing 1985; Carter and Ginsberg 1986), but other evidence suggests that errors have a suspicious tendency to result in higher reimbursement to hospitals (Hsia et al. 1988). A reabstraction study at The RAND Corporation has attempted to clarify trends. The major issue behind these studies is whether the average resource needs of hospitalized patients are actually increasing from year to year, as DRG-based data would suggest, or whether hospitals are simply becoming more adept at causing codes to creep.

The reverse of DRG creep also occurs. For example, many more patients are now assigned to DRG 410 (chemotherapy) than before DRGs were a basis for payment. This particular DRG provides rather low payment, and the change reflects aggressive definition of correct coding and policing efforts by peer review organizations.

The DRG system is in continual evolution; Medicare publishes revisions every year and variants have begun to develop.

For example, the state of New York now uses a DRG system that includes much more complex classifications for pediatric disorders than does the Medicare system. Medicare revisions have included changes in the classification of cancer of the ovary and leukemia. Medicare removed classification rules that assigned patients over and under 70 to different DRGs, because those rules were actually reducing the accuracy of payments. The classification system is relatively easy to change, and the Health Care Financing Administration has generally been receptive to documented suggestions for refinement in the system. Because new DRG definitions must use diagnostic and procedure data found in standard discharge data, they are not always easy to create; and proposals often do not produce more accurate predictions of cost when examined against actual Medicare experience. However, it is not true that HCFA avoids changes in the DRGs because they would increase Medicare costs. Changes in DRGs cannot affect total program costs because of a process called "budget neutrality," which is discussed below.

Setting DRG Payment Weights

The relative payments for different DRGs are called DRG weights or payment weights. Weights are set empirically: they reflect the relative average actual costs (as measured by adjusted charges) for each DRG for care rendered to all Medicare patients in all hospitals. When averaged across all patients in the DRG and compared to all patients in other DRGs, the relative payment weights are fair. But the payment may differ considerably from cost for individual patients, and the total payment to a hospital for its Medicare patients may differ significantly from that hospital's total costs for care of Medicare patients.

The data used to set payment weights flow slowly. The data used for setting payment weights in the federal fiscal year 1988 came from care rendered in 1985. Thus, several years will pass from the time a new technology is introduced until the cost of that new technology is reflected in higher or lower payments for the DRGs in which it is used. It will take even more time until payment weights fully reflect the cost of a new technology, because technology diffuses into practice slowly. DRG weights only reflect the costs of average care, and if only a quarter of patients in a DRG receive a new treatment, then the DRG payment weight will reflect, even after time, only a quarter of the cost of the treatment.

This delay in resetting payments to reflect experience may

explain why many hospitals consider payments for the chemotherapy DRG too low. They are based on a period when the less
expensive chemotherapy patients, who are not treated as outpatients, were receiving inpatient care, and the more expensive chemotherapy cases were not being coded into the chemotherapy
DRG. This problem will correct itself with time.

Reports that a particular DRG is uniformly profitable or
unprofitable therefore suggest three possibilities: (1) the data may
come from a biased sample of hospitals, (2) the payment weights
may not have caught up with changes in practice, or (3) the calculations are flawed. The last possibility is particularly important
because of the number of factors involved in setting PPS
payments.

Setting the Payment for a Discharge

PPS uses a number of factors to set the payment for a discharge.
The most important factors are the following:

1. The assigned DRG
2. The intensity of the hospital's teaching activity
3. Whether the hospital is located in an urban or rural area
4. The area wage index
5. The extent to which the hospital has a disproportionate
   share of poor or elderly patients.

In addition, PPS makes "outlier" payments for patients with
unusually costly or long stays in the hospital (see below). The
complexity of this payment formula has two important effects.
First, determining the fairness of the prospective payment system
by examining a few hospitals or a limited number of admissions is
very difficult. Second, cancer centers, which tend to be in high-
wage, urban teaching settings, get much higher payments than
most community hospitals would get for the same case.

Under budget neutrality, payment rates for DRGs are set in
an interdependent way so that projected average payments per
case will be the same as in the previous year, except for an "update
factor" that is intended to reflect inflation and other factors. Congress sets the update factor, which is an extremely powerful feature of cost containment under PPS. Many analysts believe that
restraints on the update factor have had more effect on hospital
finances than have either the PPS incentives for efficiency or any
inequities in the DRG system. The typical hospital's operating

margin (or "profit") on Medicare patients dropped from about 16 percent in the first year of PPS to about 6 percent four years later.

Finally, PPS payments are expected to be fair on average, but they were never expected to be highly accurate for individual cases. The variation in costs for patients in a DRG is large enough that it does not average out, even for moderate numbers of patients. Imagine a hospital with typical costs that treats 100 patients in a typical DRG each year for many years. In a third of those years that hospital could expect to have total costs for all patients in the DRG that are at least 8 percent higher or lower than payments.

Outliers: Payment for Care Rendered

The outlier payment system is a major exception to the general rule that PPS payments are independent of care actually rendered. Outlier payments are added to the DRG-based payment for cases in which cost or length of stay grossly exceeds the average for the DRG. The outlier payment system is a kind of insurance plan devised to protect hospitals and patients against the occasional very expensive hospitalization. The system protects patients as well as hospitals because it reduces the risk that the hospital will lose so much money that it will make an inappropriate discharge. The original structure of outlier payments spread payments relatively thinly over a relatively large number of cases; proposed changes will concentrate these payments on a smaller number of patients but will pay a larger fraction of costs for those patients (*Federal Register* 1988). This strategy will focus payments on such cases as acute leukemias, extreme burns, severe trauma, and other intensive extended stays.

SEVERITY OF ILLNESS

One of the most frequent complaints regarding DRG-based payments is that DRGs do not take adequate account of "severity of illness." Severity of illness is an ambiguous phrase that may refer to the degree of disease progression, the likelihood of organ system failure, a patient's acute or chronic risk of dying, the degree of current impairment, or the prospect of future impairment. The common theme is that severity refers to the likelihood that clinical features of the illness will lead to a bad outcome. The word "risk" is preferable to "severity," because it includes other sources of risk such as a decision to palliate suffering rather than preserve life.

This is a special issue for patients with advanced metastatic disease.

There are two approaches to measuring severity or risk. One is to evaluate the patient at the time of admission. Because a hospital has little control over the patient's condition at admission, it seems entirely fair to make higher payments for patients whose risk at admission makes them likely to be more expensive. A second approach is to evaluate how sick the patient becomes during the admission. This approach obviously includes the results of complications and failure to respond to treatment, and paying for this kind of severity or risk may mean paying more for treatment that is less effective. However, complications and failure to respond to therapy result in prolonged intensive care, which results in very high costs. Purists would prefer to pay only for differences present at admission, but our ability to predict complications and poor response is very poor. Thus, it is not yet clear how we should compromise between a weak measure of admission risk and a more accurate measure of total risk during the admission.

Although any hospital can get a run of unusually sick patients by chance, there are only three ways in which a hospital is likely to systematically get patients who are more severely ill on admission:

1. Screen out patients with mild illnesses, who would be admitted at other hospitals, or treat them as outpatients.

2. Serve a population in which severe illness is more prevalent or in which general health status makes patients more vulnerable to complications.

3. Receive severely ill patients by referral or transfer.

The relationship of cost to either risk or severity is complex. First, patients who die rapidly tend to have low total costs (even though their cost per day may be high). Second, cancer patients who are close to death with metastases are likely to receive only relatively inexpensive palliative therapy.

Severity is sometimes used simply as a term for clinical factors that are likely to produce high costs. DRGs do measure this kind of severity, although quite imperfectly, through the use of the principal diagnosis and additional diagnoses. The use of additional diagnoses may become substantially more sophisticated as the result of unpublished work by Jon Conklin at Systemetrics on Disease Staging and by Robert Fetter at Yale on DRGs. There are two other diagnosis-based systems of classification: patient management categories and computerized disease staging. Some years ago, they did not give substantially better prediction of costs than did DRGs (Calore and Iezzoni 1987). A more recent revision of disease staging, however, may provide an improvement in prediction of costs comparable to the improvement in DRGs that has emerged from work at Yale.

In contrast to these systems that are based on diagnostic data, a number of systems for measuring risk (including Apache, MedisGroups, Clinical Staging, and Computerized Severity Index) require abstracting physiological data and physical findings from the medical record (Knaus et al. 1985; Iezzoni, Moskowitz, and Ash 1988; Jencks and Dobson 1987; U.S. Department of Health and Human Services 1987). Such systems may be more successful in predicting death than in predicting cost of care for individual cases (Iezzoni and Moskowitz 1988; Iezzoni, Moskowitz, and Ash 1988). Medicare does not use any of these systems for payment, but HCFA is studying severity and risk adjustments carefully.

Evidence suggests that unmeasured variation in severity of illness on admission accounts for only a modest part of variation in cost among individual cases and an even smaller fraction of variation in average cost per case among hospitals (Iezzoni and Moskowitz 1988). (This finding is supported by unpublished work by Kurt Price at the Prospective Payment Assessment Commission and by Jencks at HCFA.) Thus, adding a severity measure to the DRG payment system would probably not substantially reduce the degree to which hospitals either profit or lose under PPS (U.S. Department of Health and Human Services 1987).

These findings contrast with Susan Horn's work with her Severity of Illness index, which did indicate that severity had a substantial role in interhospital cost differences (Horn, Sharkey, et al. 1985; Horn, Bulkley, et al. 1985). Because others have found Horn's earlier instrument only moderately reliable (Lloyd and Rissing 1985), and because she is no longer working to refine that instrument, the validity of her findings may never be fully resolved.

Severity and Cancer

Research on risk and cost in cancer is less extensive and the relationships are likely to be quite complex (Horn and Sharkey 1986). Severely ill cancer patients may be more likely to receive palliative care than severely ill patients with some other diseases. Cancer centers specialize in complex and unusual cases, and they often provide more extensive staging and characterization of disease, as well as more careful monitoring of therapy. It is not at all obvious, however, that these centers treat patients who are generally more severely ill than those seen in community hospitals. (Certain aggressive tumors may be concentrated in cancer centers, but most of these are easily identified by diagnosis codes, and risk/severity measures are not necessary.) From the perspective of risk/severity, the use of cancer centers as referral sites for staging and aggressive management of early disease may more than offset any referrals for near-terminal disease. A more fruitful approach to understanding the costs of cancer centers may be to consider the purpose of the admission and the intensity of the care rendered.

PURPOSE OF ADMISSION

Even more than most chronic diseases, cancer treatment has phases. Admissions with identical diagnoses and severity of illness can have very different purposes and very different costs. At best, the available data allows only inferences to the purpose of an admission, but it certainly seems likely that costs will differ for an admission for diagnosis, staging, and treatment compared to an admission for treatment when the diagnosis was already known. Likewise, costs for an admission for palliative relief of intestinal obstruction may well differ from those for curative resection with extensive efforts to remove all local and distant nodes and invasion.

INTENSITY OF CARE

There is some evidence that referral centers differ from other hospitals in the intensity of the care they provide rather than the characteristics of the patients they treat (Jencks and Bobula 1988). In cancer care, this can have two meanings. First, cancer centers may provide much more intensive diagnostic services and much more aggressive therapeutic services when complications occur. Second, there is considerable suspicion in the cancer community that physicians and centers differ extensively in how aggressively they manage similar tumors. If cancer centers provide, for example, much higher doses of chemotherapy and radiation, then they are almost certain to experience more complications of therapy, and those complications will raise costs.

If cancer centers are more expensive than less specialized facilities because of appropriate intensity of care, then reimbursement raises significant moral and policy issues. DRG-based reimbursement is based on the idea that costs for a patient with a particular illness can be inferred from the illness, and that those costs should be uniform. If costs of care in cancer centers are appropriate but higher than DRG-based payments, and costs of care in less specialized facilities are inappropriately low, the solution is not simply to raise the DRG-based payments. Although this would be fair to cancer centers, it would provide a substantial and unwarranted windfall to facilities that are undertreating their patients. The problem is that we simply do not know if cancer centers are underpaid, and we do not know whether their care is better than that of less specialized facilities.

FOUR ISSUES OF SPECIAL RELEVANCE TO CANCER

Certain issues have special importance to those interested in cancer:

Protocol Patients

Medicare rules limit payment to medically necessary treatment, which is generally interpreted to mean nonexperimental treatments. Despite some controversy around the periphery, this rule has generally not limited payment for reasonable cancer treatments, even those that push the borders of the established approaches. But many friends of research fear that treating patients under protocol is more expensive than treating according to the clinician's individual judgment, and that PPS will therefore discourage hospitals from participating in research. Whether treatment under protocol is really more expensive remains to be seen. The National Center for Health Services Research has studied the relative costs for patients on protocol and patients not on protocol in the same hospital and the same DRG. The analytic problems in such a study are formidable, because patients placed on a protocol are likely to be at a different stage in their illness than patients in the same DRG who are not on protocol.

If protocol patients do prove more expensive, a political policy decision will almost surely be necessary to determine whether the costs will be borne by the National Cancer Institute and other research programs, by hospitals, or by Medicare trust funds.

Excluded Facilities

Free-standing cancer hospitals, but not other cancer units or centers, have been excluded from the prospective payment system and thus from payments by DRG. These centers are paid on the basis of historical costs updated by an annual inflation factor. The effects of this exclusion are not known, and research has focused more on refining payment for hospitals under prospective payment than on defining a basis for excluding further facilities.

Capitation and Cancer

The Health Care Financing Administration is committed to moving the Medicare program toward prepaid arrangements in which an HMO or some similar organization arranges all necessary care to the enrolled patient in return for a prospectively set annual payment. Prepaid care presents both opportunities and problems for cancer prevention and treatment. The opportunity relates to prevention, which is discussed in the next section. The most important problem is that an HMO or similar provider faces a significant risk if it provides care that is better than average for an expensive disease such as cancer. The risk is that patients with the disease will transfer to the provider that specializes in the disease and that the provider will incur very large liabilities that are not covered by the annual payment. Conversely, the prepaid model may encourage discrimination against patients with an expensive disease such as cancer, and a provider may either discourage them from enrolling or encourage them to transfer out.

This problem should not arise if the annual payment is properly adjusted for the anticipated cost of care for such patients. Medicare pays prepaid systems an amount that is adjusted for the patient's age, sex, county of residence, and whether the patient is in a nursing home; but this payment is not adjusted for any chronic conditions. HCFA has conducted very aggressive explorations of the feasibility of adjusting payments for chronic health conditions that can be identified from the medical record.

Prevention and Medicare Payments

In general, Medicare pays only for care that is medically necessary for treatment of an illness. A patient without disease is generally deemed not to need care, so Medicare generally does not pay for preventive services. Changing that rule requires an act of Congress, such as the decision to include coverage of breast cancer screening in the Medicare Catastrophic Care Act of 1988 (P.L. 100 – 360). That decision set two important precedents:

- Breast cancer screening is the first preventive screening program to be covered (pneumococcal vaccine was covered by a special act, but is a preventive action rather than a screening service); other screening might follow.

- Congress set a dollar limit on payments for screening. This is interesting, not only because it suggests a belief that prevailing mammography fees are unreasonable, but also because it reflects a concern about total costs of screening programs. Thus, the total costs of breast cancer screening may have some effect on whether other kinds of screening will be covered in the future.

Screening is closely tied to prepaid health care. One of the traditional arguments for prepaid care is that it encourages preventive services, because the prepaid provider realizes long-term savings through prevention. There is also a marketing incentive for prepaid programs to provide preventive services, since maintaining the loyalty of healthy patients may be highly profitable. Thus, the movement to prepaid care may help to resolve the problem of covering preventive services.

PROSPECTIVE PAYMENT AND THE EFFECTIVENESS OF CARE

Many critics have suggested that PPS has had an adverse impact on quality of care and that patients are discharged "sicker and quicker." We are still not able to assess the impact of PPS on the effectiveness of medical care. Shorter hospital stays can be good for patients, as surgeons found when early ambulation averted many postoperative complications. Discharging patients before they are completely recovered may be in their interest, especially if discharge planning is efficient. Hospital-associated death rates have increased since the start of PPS, but the increase appears to be largely attributable to an increase in the average severity of illness. Overall death rates for the elderly have not risen (Eggers 1987).

Katherine Kahn et al. (1988) of The RAND Corporation have studied the impact of PPS on quality of care, but results are not yet available. Even if there are adverse effects, it would be very difficult to distinguish the effects of change, which can be disruptive to quality care, from the ultimate quality of care in a system that has become stable. A similar ambiguity clouds many studies of change. For example, Lurie et al. (1984) showed that death rates increased in patients terminated from Medi-Cal, but they could not distinguish the disruption of continuity of care from the long-term inability to gain access to quality care from a new provider.

Critics of PPS should also understand that the politically significant question is not *whether* PPS should continue but *how* it might be improved. There is simply no politically viable alternative to PPS until prepaid health care can cover a larger share of Medicare patients.

COST AND QUALITY

There is growing emphasis on effectiveness of care as a justification for cost, and this specifically means measuring outcomes of care after using severity measurement to adjust for differences in risk. Across the country, state legislatures have enacted the requirement that data be collected that will allow such comparisons, although there is some question as to how this can be done (Jencks et al. 1988). There is a rich tradition of using related comparisons to assess treatment in clinical cancer treatment trials, and outcome studies in nonresearch settings may therefore be more feasible in cancer than in other diseases.

The emerging need to justify cost through proof of effectiveness is a pervasive issue, not one created by misers at HCFA. The state laws referred to above were generally passed at the urging of business coalitions concerned with their health insurance costs. The same issues are also likely to dominate the purchasing decisions of HMOs, PPOs, and other groups that use selective contracting. Medicare, by contrast, rarely restricts its beneficiaries' choice of hospital. However, evidence regarding effectiveness will be very important if cancer centers wish to argue that they need higher payments.

AN AGENDA FOR CANCER FINANCING

Clinicians often suggest that they are caught between their obligations to their patients and the demands of utilization review coordinators. The standards of the Joint Commission on Accreditation of Healthcare Organizations, the law, and medical ethics all give the organized medical staff a critical role in this problem. The medical staff is responsible for overseeing quality of care in the hospital, and overseeing the appropriateness of recommendations from the utilization review program is an especially appropriate area on which to concentrate.

Health Services Research

Advocates for cancer research, prevention, and treatment have long been familiar with the biomedical research basis of cancer care; they are less familiar with the research foundations of payment policy. Advocates need to recognize that health services research plays a growing part in shaping payment policy and thus determining the funds available for the biomedical and clinical programs with which they are more familiar. Health services research is not free, but it is not very expensive: HCFA's budget for research grants and contracts is about $30 million. It would be prudent for those interested in cancer care to develop some of the competence in and advocacy for health services research that they already exhibit for biomedical research.

Utilization Review

In coming years, physicians, medical staff, and utilization review systems will have to learn about averages and to learn that the costs saved on the care for one patient may have to be used to pay for more costly care for another patient. Hospitals that learn to deal with these problems will prosper, while those that continue to blame the Medicare program for their failures will eventually be identified by the public as hospitals that have failed.

Outcomes Research

Those interested in cancer care are very familiar with outcomes research aimed at comparing two treatments in controlled settings. There are fewer studies, in cancer care or other care settings, of the relative performance of treatments in less controlled settings, and even fewer studies of relative performance of different providers. These studies may be controversial and painful, but they promise to be the way of the future.

Financing Prevention

The cost of screening programs may be the greatest barrier to cancer prevention. Covering screening under programs such as Medicare may rest on our ability to control the costs. In general, therefore, advocates of cancer care need to be aware and supportive of studies of the appropriate charges for such services. Studies of this kind are threatening to the alliance of physicians and others who support cancer advocacy programs, but willingness to face these issues may be vital to expanding screening programs.

New Technology

One of the problems with cost controls such as PPS is that providers feel discouraged from introducing new technology. We do not yet have evidence that shows whether the rate of technology diffusion is actually reduced, because competition leads hospitals and others to install the most advanced equipment. Nevertheless, because the costs of new technology are widely discussed, advocates of cancer care need to support studies of the effect of cost-containment strategies on innovation. The anecdotal information now available is not an adequate guide for policy.

The kind of research described in this chapter is disconcerting to traditional clinicians and advocates. Nevertheless, unless there is substantial evidence that increased funding actually leads to more effective care, it may be difficult to persuade Congress and others to provide the money that we are convinced is needed.

REFERENCES

Calore, K. A., and Iezzoni, L. (1987). "Disease Staging and PMCs: Can They Improve DRGs?" *Medical Care* 25: 724 – 37.

Carter, G., and Ginsberg, P. (1986). "Medicare Case Mix Increase." *Health Care Financing Review* 7(4): 51 – 65.

Eggers, P. W. (1987). "Prospective Payment System and Quality: Early Results and Research Strategy." *Health Care Financing Review* (Annual Supplement): 29 – 37.

Federal Register (1988), 53 (103): 19498 – 686.

Horn, S. D.; Bulkley, G.; Sharkey, P. D.; Chambers, A. F.; Horn, R. A.; and Schramm, C. J. (1985). "Interhospital Differences in Severity of Illness." *New England Journal of Medicine* 313(1): 20 – 24.

Horn, S. D., and Sharkey, P. D. (1986). "A Study of Patients in Cancer-Related DRGs." *Journal of Cancer Program Management* 1(2): 8 – 23.

Horn, S. D.; Sharkey, P. D.; Chambers, A. F.; and Horn, R. A. (1985).

"Severity of Illness Within DRGs: Impact on Prospective Payment." *American Journal of Public Health* 75(10): 1195 – 99.

Hsia, D. C.; Krushat, W. M.; Fagan, A. B.; Tebbutt, J. A.; and Kusserow, R. P. (1988). "Accuracy of Diagnostic Coding for Medicare Patients Under the Prospective Payment System." *New England Journal of Medicine* 318: 352 – 55.

Iezzoni, L. I., and Moskowitz, M. A. (1988). "A Clinical Assessment of MedisGroups." *Journal of the American Medical Association* 260(21): 3159 – 63.

Iezzoni, L. I.; Moskowitz, M. A.; and Ash, A. S. (1988). The Ability of MedisGroups and Its Clinical Variables to Predict Cost and In-Hospital Death. Boston: Boston University Medical Center.

Jencks, S. F., and Bobula, J. D. (1988). "Does Receiving Referral and Transfer Patients Make Hospitals Expensive." *Medical Care* 26(10): 948 – 58.

Jencks, S. F.; Daley, J.; Draper, D.; Thomas, N.; Lenhart, G.; and Walker, J. (1988). "Interpreting Hospital Mortality Data: The Role of Clinical Risk Adjustment." *Journal of the American Medical Association* 260(24): 3611 – 16.

Jencks, S. F., and Dobson, A. (1987). "Refining Case-Mix Adjustment: The Research Evidence." *New England Journal of Medicine* 317: 679 – 86.

Jencks, S.; Dobson, A.; Willis, P.; and Feinstein, P. H. (1984). "Evaluating and Improving the Measurement of Hospital Case Mix." *Health Care Financing Review* (Annual Supplement): 1 – 11.

Kahn, K.; Brook, R. H.; Draper, D.; Keeler, E. B.; Rubenstein, L. V.; Rogers, W. H.; and Kosecoff, J. (1988). "Interpreting Hospital Mortality Rates: How Can We Proceed?" *Journal of the American Medical Association* 260(24): 3625 – 28.

Knaus, W. A.; Draper, E. A.; Wagner, D. P.; and Zimmerman, J. E. (1985). "APACHEII: A Severity of Disease Classification System for Severely Ill Patients." *Critical Care Medicine* 13: 818 – 29.

Lloyd, S. S., and Rissing, J. P. (1985). "Physician and Coding Errors in Patient Records." *Journal of the American Medical Association* 254: 1330 – 36.

Lurie, N.; Ward, N. B.; Shapiro, M. F.; and Brook, R. H. (1984). "Termination from Medi-Cal—Does It Affect Health." *New England Journal of Medicine* 311: 480 – 84.

U.S. Department of Health and Human Services. (1987). *DRG Refinement: Outliers, Severity of Illness, and Intensity of Care*, Report to Congress. Washington, DC: U.S. Government Printing Office.

5 Reimbursement Issues in Achieving Cancer Control Objectives: Setting the Stage

Lester Breslow

ABSTRACT. While substantial efforts to combat cancer have been underway for decades, the idea of actually bringing it under some measure of control has only recently come to the fore. Unfortunately, present patterns of reimbursement for medical care do not favor achieving the objectives in cancer control. This chapter discusses several reimbursement issues including incorporation of cancer prevention and screening services into medical care reimbursement mechanisms, pricing for prevention and screening services, state-of-the-art diagnosis and treatment, and commercialization. Clarifying and resolving these key reimbursement issues will be highly important in arriving at our goals of cancer control.

Cancer control is rising to prominence on the U.S. health agenda, both because the disease is now responsible for one-fourth of the nation's deaths and because modalities for bringing down cancer mortality are now at hand. While substantial efforts to combat cancer have been underway for decades, the idea of actually bringing it under some measure of control has only recently come to the fore.

Table 5.1: Causes of Cancer Mortality

Factor or Class of Factors	Percent of All Cancer Deaths	
	Best Estimate	Range of Acceptable Estimates
Tobacco	30%	25 – 40%
Alcohol	3	2 – 4
Diet	35	10 – 70
Reproductive and sexual behavior	7	1 – 13
Occupation	4	2 – 8
Pollution	2	1 – 5
Industrial products	1	1 – 2
Medicines and medical procedures	1	0.5 – 3
Geophysical factors	3	2 – 4

Source: R. Doll and R. Peto, "The Causes of Cancer: Quantitative Estimates of Avoidable Risks of Cancer in the United States Today," *Journal of the National Cancer Institute* 66, no. 6 (1981): 1191 – 1308.

AN OVERVIEW: THE BASIS FOR CANCER CONTROL

The scientific background for the control of cancer consists of several advances. First of all, discovery of several causative factors has provided the basis for prevention. Quite widely known is the quantitative estimate of causative factors in the occurrence of cancer in the United States, which Doll and Peto made in 1981 (Table 5.1). Most significant in cancer causation, of course, is the role of cigarette smoking. Diet is also high on the list, although the quantitative aspect of that factor is less definite.

Beyond the possibilities of prevention, which are apparent in Table 5.1, technological developments in screening for cancer and in the treatment of cancer open up ways of bringing cancer under control.

Slow but steady advances in application of knowledge concerning prevention, early detection, and effective treatment of cancer have already yielded substantial gains against the disease. Mortality from cancer among young children began to decline sharply in the 1950s. By the 1960s, there was notable progress into the later childhood years, and by the 1970s into the middle years of life. Now cancer mortality seems to be declining throughout the first two-thirds of the average duration of life in our country (Table 5.2).

Table 5.2: Age-Specific Death Rates per 100,000 Population for Malignant Neoplasms, United States, Selected Years, 1950–84

Age	1950	1960	1970	1980	1982	1984
All ages, age adjusted	124.4	125.8	129.9	132.8	132.5	133.5
All ages, crude	139.8	149.2	162.8	183.9	187.2	191.8
Under 1 year	8.7	7.2	4.7	3.2	3.7	3.1
1–4 years	11.7	10.9	7.5	4.5	4.6	4.0
5–14 years	6.7	6.8	6.0	4.3	4.1	3.6
15–24 years	8.6	8.3	8.3	6.3	5.9	5.5
25–34 years	20.0	19.5	16.5	13.7	13.2	13.0
35–44 years	62.7	59.7	59.5	48.6	46.2	46.6
45–54 years	175.1	177.0	182.5	180.0	176.0	170.5
55–64 years	392.9	396.8	423.0	436.1	439.7	448.4
65–74 years	692.5	713.9	754.2	817.9	824.9	835.1
75–84 years	1,153.3	1,127.4	1,168.0	1,232.3	1,238.7	1,272.3
85 years and over	1,451.0	1,450.0	1,417.3	1,594.6	1,598.6	1,604.0

Source: U.S. Department of Health and Human Services, *Health United States 1986*, DHHS Pub. No. (PHS) 87-1232 (Washington, DC: U.S. Government Printing Office, 1987).

Experience during the past few decades, along with the anticipation of further advances in knowledge and its application, has emboldened the National Cancer Institute leadership to set as an objective for the year 2000 reducing cancer mortality by as much as 50 percent (National Cancer Institute 1986a). This goal would be achieved through the vigorous pursuit of each of the three major modalities of cancer control: prevention, screening, and treatment (Table 5.3).

Although Table 5.3 indicates objectives for the entire population, it is important to consider that we face a lag with respect to treating cancer (and essentially all health matters) among certain segments of the population in the United States. For example, cancer incidence and mortality are much higher among blacks than among whites in the United States (National Cancer Institute 1986b). Special efforts will be necessary if we are to be successful in overcoming this persistent, disgraceful situation. Another factor that needs to be addressed is the less than adequate treatment of breast cancer (and possibly other forms of cancer) among older people compared with that among younger people, even taking into account the stage of the disease and other pertinent conditions (Greenfield et al. 1987).

PROGRESS IN CANCER CONTROL

Unfortunately, present patterns of reimbursement for medical care in our country do not favor achieving the objectives of cancer control. The principal payment mechanism was designed with other aims in mind. It emphasized, first, reimbursement for hospital services; then fees for surgical procedures; and, subsequently, other medical procedures for diagnosis and treatment of disease by any licensed physician. Only recently has significant attention been given to quality, and effort in that direction has started slowly.

For decades the various elements of the dominant fee-for-service health insurance industry eschewed paying for preventive services. They avoided incorporating such services into their benefit plans on the grounds that no "risk" was involved and that insurance was supposed to protect against loss from events consequent to some "risk." Besides, it was said, people could budget for themselves for periodic prevention services, without having to add the administrative costs of insurance company processing.

Further, the health services insurance industry avoided paying for counseling services by physicians, for example, to help patients overcome tobacco addiction. On the other hand, procedures involving new mechanical technology were readily admitted to the payment system.

That was the situation until a very few years ago and, in general, it still prevails. However, a new dimension to that long-standing pattern is entering the scene. Health insurance companies are seriously exploring, and some have even initiated, payment for cancer prevention and screening services. For example, a consortium of major insurance companies sponsors the INSURE project (Logsdon 1986). That project offers, in a few fee-for-service practice situations, a substantial package of preventive services. These are based on the Lifetime Health Monitoring Program (Breslow and Somers 1977). Geared to a negotiated payment, the services include 15 minutes of counseling time regarding health risks such as tobacco and alcohol, as well as mammography and cervical cytology and other items pertinent to cancer control. Experience in the study situations is being compared to that in similar practice situations, where the preventive services are not systematically offered. Preliminary results indicate that the preventive services package is feasible in the insurance mode and effective in reducing health risks. This and other experience may

Table 5.3: Cancer Control Objectives: Summary

I. PREVENTION

Target	Rationale	Year 2000 Objective
Smoking	The causal relationship between smoking and cancer has been scientifically established.	Reduce the percentage of adults who smoke from 34 percent (in 1983) to 15 percent or less.
		Reduce the percentage of youths who smoke by age 20 from 36 percent (in 1983) to 15 percent or less.
Diet	Research indicates that high fat and low fiber consumption may increase the risk for various cancers. In 1983 the National Academy of Sciences reviewed research on diet and cancer and recommended a reduction in fat; more recent studies led the National Cancer Institute to recommend an increase in fiber. Research is underway to verify the causal relationships and to test the impact on cancer incidence.	Reduce average consumption of fat from 40 percent to 25 percent or less of total calories.
		Increase average consumption of fiber from 8–12 grams per day to 20–30 grams per day.

II. SCREENING

Target	Rationale	Year 2000 Objective
Breast	The effectiveness of breast screening in reducing mortality has been scientifically established.	Increase the percentage of women aged 50–70 who have an annual physical breast exam coupled with mammography to 80 percent from 45 percent for physical exam alone and 15 percent for mammography.
Cervix	The effectiveness of cervical screening in reducing mortality has been scientifically established.	Increase the percentage of women who have a Pap smear every 3 years to 90 percent from 79 percent (ages 20–39) and to 80 percent from 57 percent (ages 40–70).

III. TREATMENT

Target	Rationale	Year 2000 Objective
Transfer of research results to practice	NCI review of clinical trial and Surveillance, Epidemiology, and End Results (SEER) program data indicate that, for certain cancer sites, mortality in SEER is greater than mortality experienced in clinical trials.	Increase adoption of state-of-the-art treatment.

Source: P.G. Greenwald and E.J. Sendik, *Cancer Control Objectives for the Nation: 1985–2000. NCI Monographs.* no. 2 (1986): 3–76.

shift the emphasis in third-party thinking and behavior toward payment for services that would be helpful in cancer control.

Another straw in the wind is the decision by Blue Cross and Blue Shield of North Dakota to offer subscribers routine mammography screening, with a payment of $50 in 1986 acceptable to 90 percent of all physicians practicing in North Dakota (Blue Cross and Blue Shield 1987).

REIMBURSEMENT ISSUES: A DRAIN ON CANCER CONTROL

Several reimbursement issues surround the achievement of cancer control objectives through prevention, screening, and treatment. Among them is the incorporation of cancer prevention and screening services into our medical care reimbursement mechanisms. In the past, third-party payers have been extremely reluctant to accept this principle and, unfortunately, those in the cancer care community have given the matter little attention.

Seeking appropriate reimbursement for the whole battery of services that are important to cancer control would probably be more appealing to all parties concerned, and perhaps more effective. It also seems more likely to attract public support. Imagine the potential consequences if the cancer care community were to shift even one-half the energies that it now focuses on getting around the DRG specifications and similar problems to linking up reimbursement with the full spectrum of cancer control objectives. Emphasizing the narrow view—what's in it for my institution—does not seem to be winning many friends or influencing many people these days.

A second and somewhat related issue is pricing for prevention and screening services. For example, charges for a mammography in Los Angeles have ranged in recent years from $125 to $200. In special campaigns, however, the price has been brought down to $70. It is widely recognized that an efficient operation designed for breast cancer screening would actually cost considerably less than that. If we are to save the approximately 15,000 women's lives that are now lost unnecessarily to breast cancer each year, we must tackle the organization and cost issues involved. The technology to save those 15,000 lives (and another 5,000 from cervical cancer) is available and the methods have been demonstrated. Is our fundamental motive to save those lives or to preserve the present, and not too promising, pattern of financing institutions for cancer care? Pretending that these motives are identical will not wash much longer. People see the discrepancy. The motives do overlap, but institutional preservation needs to be brought into much closer alignment with the underlying social objective, cancer control.

A third reimbursement issue relates to the third modality for achieving cancer control objectives; namely, state-of-the-art diagnosis and treatment. Fee-for-service payments through third-party carriers in the United States were established and have been maintained to preserve the traditional style of medical practice. That type of medical practice has certainly accomplished much good for the health care field. The growth of prepaid group practice, however, has changed the scene. The new form of practice has emerged because of perceived inadequacies in the traditional system. Furthermore, modifications are being introduced into the fee-for-service system.

As far as cancer care is concerned, one study did not find the HMO system preferable (Greenwald 1987). The cases in that system were diagnosed somewhat earlier than in fee-for-service practice, but there was an almost compensating delay in getting them to treatment.

Hard evidence concerning the extent to which current practice provides state-of-the-art therapy for cancer is not widely available. There is some indication, however, that such therapy is applied only irregularly. For example, one study has disclosed that patients over the age of 70 received significantly less appropriate surgery for breast cancer than did patients 50 to 69 years of age, even when factors other than age were taken into account (Greenfield et al. 1987). Furthermore, physicians generally recognize considerable variation among themselves with respect to competence in dealing with cancer. Yet the reimbursement system does very little to encourage the most expert treatment available for cancer patients. Recent moves in that direction, such as paying for second opinions on proposed surgical procedures (not just for cancer), are perhaps preparing the field for a more aggressive stance toward assuring the highest achievable quality of care for cancer patients. Much remains to be done in that direction.

A fourth issue, commercialization, affects medical care generally, and the care of cancer patients in particular. Presenting the handling of cancer patients as a "product line" exemplifies the commercial spirit that is penetrating oncology (Mortenson 1986). While marketplace-type competition appears to offer some favorable incentives in medical care, adopting a dollar "bottom line" as essentially the only managerial focus will inevitably steer the management of cancer patients away from what would be best for achieving cancer control objectives. Clarifying and resolving key reimbursement issues in cancer control will be highly important in arriving at the uppermost goals shared by those of us in the cancer control community.

REFERENCES

Blue Cross and Blue Shield Association. (1987). *Consumer Exchange* (Washington, DC), January 1987.

Breslow, L., and Somers, A. R. (1977). "Lifetime Health Monitoring Program: A Practical Approach to Preventive Medicine." *New England Journal of Medicine* 296(11): 601 – 608.

Greenfield, S.; Blanco, D. M.; Elashoff, R. M.; and Ganz, P. A. (1987). "Patterns of Care Related to Age of Breast Cancer Patients." *Journal of the American Medical Association* 257(20): 2766 – 70.

Greenwald, H. (1987). "HMO Membership, Copayment and Initiation of Care for Cancer: A Study of Working Adults." *American Journal of Public Health* 77(4): 461 – 66.

Logsdon, D. N. (1986). "Should Health Insurance Cover Preventive Services?" *The Internist* 27(9): 11 – 13.

Mortenson, L. (1986). "Editorial," *Journal of Cancer Program Management* 1, no. 2 (November).

National Cancer Institute. (1986a). *Cancer Control Objectives for the Nation: 1985 – 2000.* NCI Monographs, no. 2. NIH Pub. No. 86-2880.

———. (1986b). Division of Cancer Prevention and Control. *Report of the Secretary's Task Force on Black and Minority Health.* Vol. III, Cancer. U.S. Department of Health and Human Services. Washington, DC: U.S. Government Printing Office.

Part III

Cancer Cost Issues

While Part II examined the overall economic burden of cancer, Part III turns to more specific issues regarding the cost of cancer. Under the new cost-containment programs, there is an increasing need to be able to quantify and explain the growth and distribution of cancer costs. Specific information on cancer costs can provide both a baseline against which savings can be measured and an opportunity to determine where future savings might take place. Such information is vital if we are to make decisions regarding the allocation of finite health resources and the effective use of those resources for cancer.

The Medicare program is of particular interest, since care for cancer patients has a significant impact on Medicare program expenses. The Third National Cancer Survey found that, for cancer patients over 65 years old, Medicare paid expenses in nearly 88 percent of the cases (Scotto and Chiazze 1976). Per capita Medicare expenses in the last year of life are substantially higher for persons dying of cancer than for persons dying of the other two leading causes of death, heart disease and stroke (Riley et al. 1987). Despite the importance of cancer care in understanding medical care costs, there have been relatively few studies analyzing the costs for terminally ill cancer patients and none that look at expenses for a cohort through time.

Chapter 6, written by Gerald Riley and James Lubitz of the Health Care Financing Administration, takes an important step toward filling this gap in knowledge. Retrospectively examining Medicare claims data, Riley and Lubitz found that per capita costs for cancer decedents in the last year of life were 6.6 times higher than the average for all beneficiaries. Expenses for cancer decedents in the last year of life declined sharply with age, with expenses for those 85 years old and older considerably lower than those for younger decedents.

Similar results for the nonelderly population were found by James O. Gibbs, Robert D. Narkiewicz, and Janice M. Moore of Blue Cross and Blue Shield, who discuss their study of terminal cancer in Chapter 7. They found that hospital use and costs escalate rapidly in the last few months of life and vary considerably by geographic area, suggesting that potential exists for cost savings. They explore the potential for new third-party efforts to reduce costs through cost management and managed care programs, including increases in cost sharing, second surgical opinion programs, benefit changes, preadmission review, alternative delivery systems, and hospice benefits. They suggest that managed care programs have good potential for reducing the high costs associated with terminal cancer care.

Chapter 8, written by Mary S. Baker, Larry G. Kessler, and Robert C. Smucker, continues the examination of cancer costs by looking at the lifetime costs of cancer. It is the lifetime cost of treatment that could be eliminated or reduced by effective cancer control programs. By dividing treatment costs into initial treatment, continuing care, and terminal care phases, the authors are able to compare costs by phase and cancer site. This information is important in determining the potential savings in treatment costs as a result of cost-effective planning of cancer-related health care activities.

The final chapter in this part was written by Stuart O. Schweitzer of the University of California, Los Angeles. Schweitzer notes that the economic burden of cancer is a function of two factors: incidence and costs. He develops an interesting and important methodology to calculate the changing burden of cancer by focusing on changing patterns of disease. By analyzing the costs of cancer treatment by site, we can identify those cancer sites where significant gains can be achieved through cancer control measures, such as prevention through changing health behaviors. He concludes that, although much of the cancer cost story is bleak, potential for improvement is within our reach.

REFERENCES

Riley, G.; Lubitz, J.; Prihoda, R.; and Rabey, E. (1987). "Use and Costs of Medicare Services by Cause of Death." *Inquiry* 24(Fall): 233 – 44.

Scotto, J., and Chiazze, L. (1976). *Third National Cancer Survey: Hospitalizations and Payments to Hospitals, Part A: Summary.* U.S. Department of Health, Education, and Welfare. DHEW Pub. No. (NIH) 76-1094. Washington, DC: U.S. Government Printing Office.

6 Longitudinal Patterns in Medicare Costs for Cancer Decedents

Gerald F. Riley and James Lubitz

ABSTRACT. To study longitudinal patterns of cancer care, death certificate information was linked to six calendar years of Medicare claims data for aged beneficiaries who died of cancer in 1979. We found per capita costs for cancer decedents in the last calendar year of life were 6.6 times higher than the average for all beneficiaries. Expenses were above average even in the fourth calendar year before death. Over a six-year period before death, the most costly cancers among those we studied were bladder cancer, female breast cancer, and leukemia, and costs were positively related to survival time. Expenses of cancer decedents in the last years of life declined sharply with age, with expenses for those 85 and over considerably lower than those for younger decedents.

The care of terminally ill cancer patients has a significant impact on the expenses of the Medicare program. Per capita Medicare expenses in the last year of life are substantially higher for persons dying of cancer than for persons dying of the other two leading causes of death—heart disease and stroke (Riley et al. 1987). Despite the importance of cancer care for understanding medical care costs, there have been relatively few studies analyzing the costs for terminally ill cancer patients and none looking at expenses for a cohort through time.

The study by Riley et al. cited above looked at Medicare costs in the last year of life for persons dying of cancer in 1979. It found that cancer decedents averaged $8,000 in the last 12 months of life compared to $5,200 for all decedents. There was relatively little variation in expenses among four specific types of cancer studied. A study by Long et al. (1984) looked at the medical care charges for three types of cancer for terminally ill patients under 65 years of age in the last 12 months of life, using claims data from Blue Cross and Blue Shield plans in three states. They found mean charges of $21,200 in 1980 dollars during the last 12 months of life, of which inpatient hospital charges constituted 73 percent of the total. Mor and Kidder (1985) looked at expenses of a sample of terminally ill Medicare cancer patients who died between October 1980 and December 1983 and received care in either home-based hospices, hospital-based hospices, or conventional care settings. They found that conventional care patients averaged $14,800 in Medicare expenses in the last year of life, excluding physician services costs, which were estimated to be 10 to 15 percent of the total. Hospice care patients were less expensive, on average. (The differences in expenses reported in the three studies are due to differences in prices in the different geographic areas studied, differences in what services were included, and whether costs or charges were examined.)

The previous studies have two important limitations for studying the costs of care for persons dying of cancer—they look at costs only in the last year of life and they break out costs separately only for a few types of cancer. Many cancer patients undergo a lengthy period of illness and treatment that can extend for many years before death. Consequently, medical services received in the last year of life may represent only a portion of the total care received during the entire course of treatment, and examining patterns of care only for the most common cancer types may overlook important differences found in less common types of cancer. This chapter extends previous work on the costs of terminal cancer care by examining the medical care costs of cancer decedents over their last six years of life. This will provide a more comprehensive picture of the total impact on Medicare expenditures of care rendered to beneficiaries who die of cancer. The following questions are addressed in this chapter:

- At what point before death do beneficiaries begin to receive higher than average amounts of services?
- How much and what kinds of services do they receive as they approach the year of death?
- Do the quantity and mix of services differ by type of cancer?

- What is the dollar impact on the Medicare program of care rendered to cancer decedents in their last year and last two years of life?

METHODS

The study population was selected from a 5 percent national probability sample of aged Medicare beneficiaries who died in 1979. These decedents were identified from the health insurance master (HIM) file, which contains demographic and entitlement information and date of death, if applicable, for every Medicare beneficiary. The sample of decedents was selected on the basis of their Medicare identification numbers.

In order to obtain information on underlying cause of death for these decedents, we first arranged for a link of the Health Care Financing Administration 5 percent sample to the national death index (NDI), maintained by the National Center for Health Statistics (NCHS). The NDI contains the death certificate numbers for all deaths in the United States since 1979; it does not contain cause of death information, however. Using the death certificate number obtained from the NDI, the sample was next linked to the mortality statistics file (also maintained by NCHS), which contains cause of death information, as well as death certificate numbers. Cause of death was ultimately obtained for 58,382 individuals, or 92 percent of the aged decedents in the sample.

Once cause of death information was obtained from the mortality statistics file, the sample was then linked to the continuous Medicare history sample file (CMHSF) to obtain a complete record of the Medicare reimbursement and utilization experience for these decedents. The CMHSF is a 5 percent longitudinal research file, with sample selection based on the last two digits of the beneficiary's Medicare number. New enrollees whose Medicare numbers place them in the sample are added to the file, and the records of enrollees who die are retained. The file contains demographic and entitlement information, and information on the use of Medicare-covered services. Included is summary information on annual use of physician, hospital outpatient, and home health services, and selected information on all inpatient hospital and skilled nursing facility (SNF) stays. Using this longitudinal file, we were able to track Medicare utilization and expenses retrospectively to 1974 for individuals who died in 1979. For this study, we selected persons whose underlying cause of death was "malignant neoplasms, including neoplasms of lymphatic and hemapoietic tissues" (ICD-9-CM codes 140 – 208). This yielded a sample of 11,469 persons.

All cost and utilization data are summarized by calendar year. Consequently, decedents had, on average, only six months of program exposure in 1979, whereas comparison group members (described below) averaged 12 months. An earlier study estimated that 77 percent of costs in the last year of life occur in the last six months (Lubitz and Prihoda 1984).

One percent samples of all aged persons entitled to Medicare in each of the years from 1974 to 1979 were selected from the CMHSF to serve as comparison groups. This selection of annual cross-sectional samples of aged beneficiaries allowed us to compare decedent reimbursements for specific years before death to average program expenses for each of those years. This was done by forming ratios of average reimbursements for beneficiaries dying of specific causes to average reimbursements for all aged beneficiaries in a given year. These ratios will be referred to as reimbursement ratios. A reimbursement ratio above 1 indicates that per capita expenses for a given cause of death were above the average for all Medicare beneficiaries in a given year.

The data are limited to Medicare-covered services and Medicare reimbursements for these services. Part A (Hospital Insurance) of Medicare covers hospital, skilled nursing facility, and home health agency (HHA) services; Part B (Supplementary Medical Insurance) covers physician and other medical, hospital outpatient, and some HHA services. Services of importance to the aged that are not covered by Medicare are nursing home care below the skilled level and outpatient prescription drugs. These services are mostly paid by the Medicaid program, by "Medigap" supplemental insurance policies, or by the beneficiaries themselves. Beginning in 1991, Medicare will provide coverage of outpatient prescription drugs under the Medicare Catastrophic Coverage Act of 1988.

RESULTS

Use of Services

About 230,000 aged Medicare beneficiaries died of cancer in 1979—18 percent of all aged decedents in that year. Thirty-one percent of cancer decedents had cancer of the digestive organs or

Table 6.1: Sample Size and Percent of Aged Medicare Cancer Decedents, by Type of Cancer, 1979

Type of Cancer	ICD-9-CM Code(s)	Sample Size	Percent
All cancers	140–208	11,469	100%
Digestive organs and peritoneum	150–159	3,506	31
Stomach	151	494	4
Colon	153	1,469	13
Pancreas	157	640	6
Trachea, bronchus, and lung	162	2,548	22
Female breast	174	733	6
Prostate	185	975	9
Bladder	188	349	3
Leukemia	204–208	443	4

Source: Continuous Medicare history sample file (CMHSF) from the Health Care Financing Administration linked with the mortality statistics file from the National Center for Health Statistics.

Note: Excludes end-stage renal disease beneficiaries.

peritoneum as the underlying cause of death, including 13 percent of the total who died of colon cancer (Table 6.1). Cancer of the lung, trachea, or bronchus was the cause of death for 22 percent of the sample.

Reimbursement ratios for all covered services indicate that cancer decedents had expenses 6.64 times above the average in the calendar year of death (Table 6.2). This varied somewhat by type of cancer, ranging from 5.59 for cancer of the prostate to 7.80 for cancer of the bladder. All other reimbursement ratios in the calendar year of death were between 6.10 and 6.95. Expenses were also very high in the second to last calendar year; for all cancer decedents, costs were 3.91 times above the average. For the third to last year and earlier, average expenses were considerably lower. They were below the program average (reimbursement ratio of .90) in the sixth to last calendar year, probably because the comparison group included beneficiaries who died that year (and presumably incurred high costs), whereas the cancer group were all survivors by definition, since they did not die until 1979. The patterns of expenses over time varied considerably by type of cancer. Persons dying of stomach and pancreatic cancer incurred costs below the average in the fourth to last calendar year and earlier. This undoubtedly reflects the relatively brief survival time for these groups of patients following diagnosis. On the other

Table 6.2: Reimbursement Ratios for 1979 Aged Medicare Cancer Decedents: All Covered Services, by Type of Cancer, 1974–79

Type of Cancer	6th to Last Year	5th to Last Year	4th to Last Year	3rd to Last Year	2nd to Last Year	Last Year	Six Years Combined
All cancers	0.90	1.03	1.29	1.81	3.91	6.64	2.90
Digestive organs	0.85	0.91	1.22	1.84	3.78	6.65	2.82
Stomach	0.74	0.90	0.82	1.44	3.06	6.76	2.56
Colon	0.92	1.05	1.58	2.23	4.24	6.28	2.98
Pancreas	0.77	0.74	0.85	1.37	3.32	6.76	2.56
Lung	0.83	0.93	1.10	1.34	3.51	6.55	2.76
Female breast	1.09	1.21	1.78	2.46	4.30	6.10	3.14
Prostate	1.06	1.26	1.35	2.10	3.68	5.59	2.69
Bladder	1.33	1.80	2.00	3.03	5.78	7.80	3.87
Leukemia	1.14	1.05	1.53	2.12	3.83	6.95	3.01

Source: Continuous Medicare history sample file (CMHSF) from the Health Care Financing Administration linked with the mortality statistics file from the National Center for Health Statistics.
Note: Excludes end-stage renal disease beneficiaries.

hand, bladder cancer decedents, who had the highest reimbursement ratios in each year, had expenses one-third higher than the
program average in the sixth year before death. This is consistent
with the relatively long survival times after diagnosis of this condition, during which time the patients usually receive medical
treatment.

For the years 1974–79 combined, the highest per capita
expenses were attributable to cancers of the bladder and breast,
both of which exhibited high reimbursement ratios for several
years before death. An interesting contrast in patterns of care over
the six-year period is provided from reimbursement data on cancers of the breast and stomach. The annual reimbursement ratios
for breast cancer decedents exceeded 1.0 in each of the six years
before death, whereas the reimbursement ratio for stomach cancer decedents does not exceed 1.0 until the third calendar year
before death. The annual reimbursement ratios for breast cancer
are greater than those for stomach cancer for all but the last year.
Undoubtedly, these patterns reflect differences in survival times
after diagnosis for the two types of cancer. During the period
1973–79, the five-year survival rate for white breast cancer
patients over 65 years of age in selected geographic areas was 53
percent; for stomach cancer, the rate was 8 percent (Ries, Pollack,
and Young 1983). Despite higher costs in the final year for stomach cancer (reimbursement ratios of 6.76 versus 6.10), costs over
the six-year study period were 18 percent lower for stomach cancer (combined reimbursement ratios of 2.56 versus 3.14). The
longer survival times for breast cancer, and the consequent need
for medical attention over a longer period, result in higher total
Medicare costs, even though costs for stomach cancer decedents
are higher in the last calendar year of life. Table 6.3 and Figure 6.1
indicate that higher expenses are associated with longer survival
times for seven common types of cancer.

The intense use of hospital services by cancer patients in the
last year of life is demonstrated by the high reimbursement ratios
for inpatient hospital services and high hospitalization rates
(Tables 6.4 and 6.5). Cancer decedents used hospital services at
the rate of 7.70 times the average in their last calendar year, ranging from 6.47 for cancer of the prostate to 8.91 for cancer of the
bladder (Table 6.4). By contrast, reimbursement ratios for physician and outpatient services averaged 4.29 in the last year. In the
second to last year, however, reimbursement ratios for inpatient
hospital services and for physician and outpatient services tended
to be very similar (3.94 and 3.97, respectively, for all cancer dece-

Table 6.3: Five-Year Survival Rates and Reimbursement Ratios
for Aged Cancer Decedents, by Type of Cancer

Type of Cancer	Survival Rate (5 Year)[a]	Reimbursement Ratios (Last 6 Years)[b]
All Cancers	28%	2.90
Stomach	8	2.56
Colon	32	2.98
Pancreas	1	2.56
Lung	7	2.76
Breast	53	3.14
Prostate	39	2.69
Bladder	42	3.87

Source: Continuous Medicare history sample file (CMHSF) from the Health
Care Financing Administration linked with the mortality statistics file from the
National Center for Health Statistics.
  [a]Based on 1973–79 data adapted from L. Ries, E. Pollack, and J. Young,
"Cancer Patient Survival: Surveillance, Epidemiology, and End Results Program,
1973–79," *Journal of the National Cancer Institute* 70, no. 4 (April 1983):
693–707.
  [b]Based on data for 1979 decedents.

dents), indicating a less intensive use of inpatient hospital services. Bladder cancer decedents used more hospital services than
other cancer decedents for each of the sixth to second calendar
years before death. For the sixth through third calendar years
before death, cancer decedents used physician and outpatient services relatively more heavily than inpatient hospital services.
Even in the sixth year before death, patients with breast, prostate,
and bladder cancers and leukemia used higher than average
amounts of physician and outpatient services.

Eighty-six percent of all cancer decedents were hospitalized
in their last calendar year (Table 6.5). Fifty-two percent were hospitalized in the second to last calendar year, ranging from 46 percent (stomach and pancreas) to 71 percent (bladder).

Use of Services by Age

Medicare expenses in the last 12 months of life have been found to
decline with increasing age for most major causes of death, with
the pattern most pronounced at the older ages (Riley et al. 1987).
Table 6.6 shows that the pattern of lower expenses for the oldest
cancer decedents persists for several years prior to the year of
death. Persons 85 and over had the lowest average expenses in the

Figure 6.1: Relationship Between Five-Year Survival and
Five-Year Reimbursement Ratio by Cancer Site

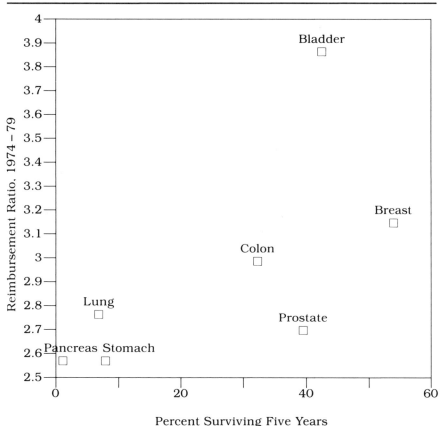

Percent Surviving Five Years

fourth to last calendar year before death, with the difference in
expenses widening as the final year approached. For example, in
the second to last calendar year, those dying at age 85 or older
averaged $2,000, versus $3,460 for those 75 to 84 and $3,883 for
those 65 to 74. The pattern of lower expenses for older decedents
was evident only for the last two calendar years of life among lung
cancer decedents, however.

The impact of age on per capita expenses among cancer decedents is shown graphically in Figure 6.2. The graph pools
inflation-adjusted expenses over the last three calendar years of
life and plots them by age at death. From age 67 to age 76

Table 6.4: Reimbursement Ratios for 1979 Aged Medicare Cancer Decedents: Inpatient Hospital and Outpatient and Physician Services, by Type of Cancer, 1974–79

Type of Cancer	6th to Last Year	5th to Last Year	4th to Last Year	3rd to Last Year	2nd to Last Year	Last Year
All cancers						
Inpatient	0.85	0.98	1.25	1.77	3.94	7.70
Physician and outpatient	1.11	1.23	1.49	2.01	3.97	4.29
Digestive organs						
Inpatient	0.82	0.87	1.21	1.85	3.88	7.75
Physician and outpatient	1.02	1.06	1.33	1.90	3.72	4.24
Stomach						
Inpatient	0.71	0.89	0.79	1.39	3.07	7.94
Physician and outpatient	0.92	1.05	0.97	1.62	3.40	4.31
Colon						
Inpatient	0.91	1.02	1.58	2.25	4.34	7.29
Physician and outpatient	1.05	1.14	1.64	2.30	4.14	3.94
Pancreas						
Inpatient	0.69	0.68	0.80	1.39	3.46	7.93
Physician and outpatient	1.05	0.94	1.06	1.37	3.23	4.54

Lung						
Inpatient	0.77	0.90	1.06	1.30	3.47	7.49
Physician and outpatient	1.04	1.07	1.28	1.56	3.83	4.64
Female breast						
Inpatient	1.01	1.07	1.66	2.21	4.20	7.01
Physician and outpatient	1.41	1.68	2.26	3.12	4.57	3.73
Prostate						
Inpatient	1.00	1.20	1.27	2.08	3.63	6.47
Physician and outpatient	1.29	1.56	1.71	2.34	3.86	3.51
Bladder						
Inpatient	1.18	1.79	1.96	3.02	5.86	8.91
Physician and outpatient	1.89	2.02	2.30	3.39	6.01	5.24
Leukemia						
Inpatient	1.07	0.96	1.51	2.20	4.06	8.46
Physician and outpatient	1.39	1.34	1.60	1.94	3.38	3.93

Source: Continuous Medicare history sample file (CMHSF) from the Health Care Financing Administration linked with the mortality statistics file from the National Center for Health Statistics.

Note: Excludes end-stage renal disease beneficiaries.

Table 6.5: Percent Hospitalized Among 1979 Aged Medicare Cancer Decedents, by Type of Cancer, 1974–79

Type of Cancer	6th to Last Year	5th to Last Year	4th to Last Year	3rd to Last Year	2nd to Last Year	Last Year
All cancers	20%	22%	25%	32%	52%	86%
Digestive organs	18	19	23	30	50	87
Stomach	17	20	19	27	46	86
Colon	18	21	27	35	54	85
Pancreas	19	17	20	23	46	90
Lung	18	19	22	27	48	87
Female breast	23	27	34	40	56	81
Prostate	22	27	30	40	59	82
Bladder	29	33	38	49	71	89
Leukemia	25	22	28	34	51	91

Source: Continuous Medicare history sample file (CMHSF) from the Health Care Financing Administration linked with the mortality statistics file from the National Center for Health Statistics.

Note: Excludes end-stage renal disease beneficiaries.

Table 6.6: Reimbursements per Enrollee for 1979 Aged Medicare Cancer Decedents, for Selected Types of Cancer, by Age, 1974–79 (adjusted for inflation)

Age at Death	6th to Last Year	5th to Last Year	4th to Last Year	3rd to Last Year	2nd to Last Year	Last Year
All Cancers						
65–74	$605	$718	$1,104	$1,638	$3,883	$6,956
75–84	712	921	1,122	1,655	3,460	6,024
85 and over	709	727	1,013	1,411	2,500	4,430
Digestive Organs						
65–74	$480	$657	$1,110	$1,718	$3,837	$6,906
75–84	703	754	1,037	1,699	3,375	6,234
85 and over	723	745	919	1,311	2,408	4,631
Lung						
65–74	$549	$578	$897	$1,087	$3,188	$6,679
75–84	659	897	971	1,305	3,252	5,507
85 and over	767	750	944	1,456	2,214	4,310

Source: Continuous Medicare history sample file (CMHSF) from the Health Care Financing Administration linked with the mortality statistics file from the National Center for Health Statistics.
Note: Excludes end-stage renal disease beneficiaries.

Figure 6.2: Average Medicare Expenses in the Last Three
Calendar Years for Cancer Decedents by Age

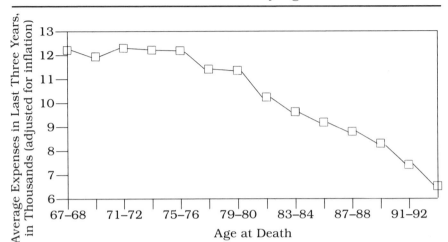

expenses vary only slightly, averaging about $12,000. After age
76, they decline sharply. For persons dying at age 85 or 86, for
example, expenses averaged only about $9,000.

The pattern of lower expenses at older ages may be explained
in part by survival times—survival time is shorter for older age
groups, among the elderly within cancer type (Ries, Pollack, and
Young 1983). The oldest cancer patients may often succumb more
quickly to the disease than their younger counterparts because of
their greater physical frailty and more frequent presence of co-
morbid conditions. Very elderly cancer patients may be unable to
withstand aggressive (and often expensive) treatments that may
be applied to younger persons. There may also be some reluctance
on the part of physicians and patients to apply "heroic" measures
to the very elderly.

Distribution of Six-Year Expenses

The distribution of expenses over the last six calendar years of life
shows substantial variation in reimbursements per person (Table
6.7).[1] Seven percent incurred over $30,000 in expenses in their
last six years (beneficiaries dying at age 70 or earlier usually had
less than six years of exposure). Forty-seven percent of decedents
had $10,000 or less in expenses. As expected, the types of cancer

Table 6.7: Percent Distribution of Medicare Expenses in the Last Six Years of Life for 1979 Aged Medicare Cancer Decedents, by Type of Cancer (adjusted for inflation)

Type of Cancer	Total	$0 – 10,000	$10,000 – 20,000	$20,000 – 30,000	Over $30,000
All cancers	100%	47%	34%	12%	7%
Digestive organs	100	48	34	12	6
Stomach	100	54	30	10	5
Colon	100	44	36	14	7
Pancreas	100	53	32	8	7
Lung	100	52	33	11	5
Female breast	100	47	31	14	8
Prostate	100	45	37	13	6
Bladder	100	27	36	21	15
Leukemia	100	46	31	13	10

Source: Continuous Medicare history sample file (CMHSF) from the Health Care Financing Administration linked with the mortality statistics file from the National Center for Health Statistics.

Note: Excludes end-stage renal disease beneficiaries.

associated with consistently high expenses were also associated with greater numbers of high cost beneficiaries. For example, nearly 15 percent of bladder cancer decedents incurred over $30,000 in expenses and only 27 percent incurred $10,000 or less. Relatively large percentages of persons dying of leukemia and breast cancer also incurred more than $30,000 in their last six years (10 and 8 percent, respectively).

SUMMARY

Medical care received by persons who die of cancer has a large impact on Medicare expenditures that extends well beyond the terminal phase of the illness. Average expenses for cancer decedents were 80 percent above the average in the third to last calendar year of life, and 30 percent above the average in the fourth to last calendar year. For certain types of cancer, higher than average costs were evident for a longer period of time; for example, expenses attributable to bladder cancer decedents were one-third higher than average in the sixth year before death. Naturally, the types of cancer that have the greatest absolute impact on Medicare costs are the most common cancers (e.g., those of the lung and colon).

The types of cancer that resulted in the highest per capita

costs were those associated with the longest survival times. The relative costliness of various types of cancer is also affected by the age distribution of the patients; expenses in the last three calendar years of life were shown to decline sharply with age for deaths occurring after age 75. Despite the fact that many cancer decedents incurred high costs for several years before death, the major financial impact occurred in the year of death, and average expenses in the last year tended to be similar among the various cancer types.

The data presented here do not, of course, yield a precise estimate of the total impact of cancer care on Medicare expenditures. For example, not all medical expenses incurred in the last few years of life are attributable directly to cancer care. On the other hand, some beneficiaries receive treatment for cancer but die of other causes, and therefore were not included in our study.

DISCUSSION

Because of the high average costs of cancer cases and the fact that cancer is a frequent cause of death among the elderly, it is not surprising that cancer care has a substantial impact on Medicare expenditures. In a 1988 report, estimates were made for the percent of annual Medicare expenditures associated with care rendered in the last 12 months and last 24 months of life for beneficiaries dying of the three major causes of death: heart disease, cancer, and stroke (Riley and Lubitz 1988). The estimates included average expenses incurred in the last 12 and 24 months of life, and not just expenses in the last calendar year(s). Annual expenditures for the care of cancer patients in their last year comprised 8.0 percent of Medicare expenses for the aged;[2] when expenses for cancer decedents who were in their second to last year were added in, the figure rose to 10.7 percent. By comparison, 9.2 percent of annual Medicare expenditures went to heart disease decedents in their last 12 months and 13.0 percent went to heart disease decedents who were in their last 24 months of life. Although reimbursements attributable to heart disease decedents account for a slightly larger portion of Medicare expenditures than those attributable to cancer decedents, the number of aged beneficiaries dying of heart disease is much greater than the number dying of cancer (41 percent of decedents versus 18 percent). The reason that Medicare spends nearly as much in total on cancer decedents as on heart disease decedents is that average costs of cancer decedents are so much greater. In their last year of life, persons dying of cancer account for approximately twice the Medicare reimbursements, on average, of persons dying of heart disease (Riley et al. 1987).

The level of Medicare program expenditures in the future may be significantly affected by trends in the incidence of various types of cancer. The National Cancer Institute has estimated that, during the period 1974 – 1983, cancer incidence rates increased among the 65 and older population at an average rate of over 1 percent per year for both males and females (National Cancer Institute 1985). Much of this increase was due to a significant increase in the incidence of cancer of the lung and bronchus, although in 1983 a significant decrease occurred for white males for the first time. Incidence of cancer of the prostate, which occurs primarily in the 65 and older age group, increased significantly between 1974 and 1983, but the increase in mortality (per 100,000 population) from this condition was not as great. Mortality for all sites combined increased over that time period for both males and females over 65 years of age. If the increase in incidence and mortality persist, Medicare expenditures would be expected to increase over time.

Trends in survival rates for cancer may also affect Medicare expenditure levels. The National Cancer Institute (1985) reported that relative survival rates rose somewhat for whites for the period 1977 – 1982, compared to 1973 – 1976. Five-year relative survival rates for colon, lung and bronchus, prostate, and bladder cancer all rose during that period. The effect of increased survival rates on expenditures is not clear. To the extent that increased survival rates reflect earlier detection and cure, expenses would decrease. Improved survival means many people may be cured and never show up at all in expense data for cancer decedents. In addition, if cancer patients die at more advanced ages, their expenses in the last few years of life should be lower than if they had died earlier. On the other hand, to the extent that patients survive longer after diagnosis and may receive treatments over a longer period of time, expenses would be expected to increase. The meaning of the data showing improved survival has been debated (Bailar and Smith 1986). To the extent that it reflects earlier diagnosis rather than improved outcome, it raises the possibility that costs may increase with no benefit in lowered mortality.

The cost of cancer reflects the incidence of the disease, costs of specific therapies, survival times, and technological advances. Recent trends in the incidence and survival after diagnosis for different cancer types, and changes in recommended therapies for certain cancers (such as for breast cancer), make clear the importance of further study to relate these factors to costs of treatment.

NOTES

1. Expenses were inflation-adjusted to 1979 dollars using the Medical Care Component of the consumer price index (CPI).
2. The numbers presented here on the percent of Medicare expenses attributable to care rendered in the last year of life are slightly higher than those presented by Riley et al. (1987) in Table 6.1 due to the different estimation methods used. The availability of multi-year data on a calendar year basis for the later report (Riley and Lubitz 1988) permits more accurate estimation of Part B expenses for specific months than was possible using the data available for the earlier article. The estimation methods are described in Riley and Lubitz (1988).

REFERENCES

Bailar, J., and Smith, E. (1986). "Progress against Cancer?" *New England Journal of Medicine* 314(19): 1226–32.

Long, S.; Gibbs, J.; Crozier, J.; Cooper, D. I., Jr.; Newman, J. F., Jr.; and Larsen, A. M. (1984). "Medical Expenditures of Terminal Cancer Patients During the Last Year of Life." *Inquiry* 21(4): 315–27.

Lubitz, J., and Prihoda, R. (1984). "The Use and Costs of Medicare Services in the Last Two Years of Life." *Health Care Financing Review* 5(3): 117–31.

Mor, V., and Kidder, D. (1985). "Cost Savings in Hospice: Final Results of the National Hospice Study." *Health Services Research* 20(4): 408–22.

National Cancer Institute. (1985). *1985 Annual Cancer Statistics Review.* U.S. Department of Health and Human Services. Bethesda, MD: National Cancer Institute.

Ries, L.; Pollack, E.; and Young, J. (1983). "Cancer Patient Survival: Surveillance, Epidemiology, and End Results Program, 1973–79." *Journal of the National Cancer Institute* 70, no. 4 (April): 693–707.

Riley, G., and Lubitz, J. (1988). "Longitudinal Patterns of Medicare Use by Cause of Death." Draft Report. Health Care Financing Administration.

Riley, G.; Lubitz, J.; Prihoda, R.; and Rabey, E. (1987). "Use and Costs of Medicare Services by Cause of Death." *Inquiry* 24(3): 233–44.

7 Managing the Cost of Terminal Cancer in the Nonelderly Population

James O. Gibbs, Robert D. Narkiewicz, and Janice M. Moore

ABSTRACT. This chapter reviews the costs and treatment of terminal cancer among the nonelderly and explores the potential impact of new third-party cost-control efforts to reduce these costs. A study of terminal cancer costs in a traditionally insured population showed that hospital use and costs escalate rapidly in the last few months of life and vary considerably by geographic area, suggesting that potential exists for cost savings. A comparison of hospice and conventional care costs found that hospice program costs were considerably lower for the last month of life, but it is concluded that significant savings will not be realized until hospice programs achieve greater control over the use of hospital days prior to the last month of life. Managed care programs appear to have good potential for reducing the high costs associated with terminal cancer care. The application of a number of these programs, including individual case management, is discussed.

The costs of terminal cancer care are a significant part of the total health care expenditures for both the elderly and nonelderly populations. This chapter will review the comparative costs and treatment of terminal cancer among the nonelderly and explore the potential impact of new third-party cost-control efforts in reducing these costs. In the last five years, purchasers and insurers have frequently altered traditional insurance products and the way they are administered in order to lower costs. Most of these efforts center on increasing deductibles and copayments, adding hospice and other benefits believed to lower costs, and imposing direct controls through managed care and preadmission review. The cost-containment potential of these alternatives varies greatly.

Interventions in the health care delivery system should be guided by knowledge and research. Unfortunately, the costs of terminal cancer care in the nonelderly population have received relatively little study. In contrast, there are numerous studies that assess the costs of such care for the population of people over 65. Even in studies that span both populations, the results are often less clear or not statistically reliable for people under 65. The reasons for this difference are clear. There are many more deaths and more cancer deaths in those over 65, and the Medicare statistical files provide a single point of access to data on much of the cost of health care for the elderly. Of the 453,492 deaths due to malignant neoplasms of all types in 1984, 291,362 or about 65 percent occurred in the elderly population. Cancer deaths were about 20 percent of all deaths in people over 65 in 1984 and about 26 percent of all deaths under 65 (National Center for Health Statistics 1986). Thus the number of terminal cancer cases in patients under age 65, although fewer than the number of cases in patients over 65, is large enough to warrant investigation of cost and treatment patterns to guide cost-containment efforts.

EXPENDITURES UNDER TRADITIONAL INSURANCE PROGRAMS

A Blue Cross and Blue Shield Association analysis of the costs for terminal care remains the only large systematic study of the costs of conventional care for terminal cancer patients under age 65 (Gibbs and Newman 1982). Data for this study were obtained from the claims records and membership files of three Blue Cross and Blue Shield Plans: Michigan, Indiana, and Georgia. The use of data from three different states allowed for some investigation of geographic differences in utilization and expenditures patterns. Cases were included where death occurred between January 1, 1978 and December 31, 1979. A retrospective definition of terminal illness was used.

All selected cases had at least one hospital inpatient claim record during the last six months of life with a diagnosis of malignant neoplasm at one of the following sites: breast; trachea, bronchus, and lung; large intestine (except rectum); or rectum and rectosigmoid junction. During the period of study, these diagnoses accounted for approximately one-half of all deaths from cancer (American Cancer Society 1980, 1981). To maximize the proportion of total medical costs captured by the claims records, only those persons who had comprehensive benefit coverage for both institutional and medical-surgical services were selected. All elderly (65 years and older) persons were excluded from the study because Medicare reimbursements were not included in these claims data.

The 1,054 persons (cases) selected made a total of 89,771 claims, representing $21.3 million in health care spending. There were 678 cases in Michigan, 340 in Indiana, and 36 in Georgia/Atlanta. For purposes of analysis, claims files were aggregated to create a summary record for each person. Complete data for the last six months of life were available for all cases, whereas there were data for only 662 cases for a full year before death.

RESULTS

Mean medical care expenditures by this sample of terminal cancer patients during their last year of life are shown in Table 7.1. Means are presented for each of the last six months of life, as well as for the last six months and last year inclusively. Total expenditures for the last year of life average $21,219 (SD $\pm$ $14,603). Spending rises at an increasing rate as the patient approaches death, with $9,375 (or 4 percent of the total) spent during the last two months and $6,161 (or 29 percent) during the final month alone.

Patterns by Type of Service

The distribution of expenditures by service category is also presented in Table 7.1. Hospital inpatient services account for the largest share of expenditures throughout the period. The hospital expenditures averaged $15,594 (SD $\pm$ $12,233) during the last year of life. The probability of hospitalization increased sharply from only .25 at six months prior to death to .94 in the last month.

The large increase in the hospital proportion of expenditures is due almost entirely to the increases in utilization, both in terms of the rate of hospitalization and the length of stay, which increased from 10 days in the last six months to 16 days in the last month (not shown in Table 7.1). Intensity of services as reflected in the Michigan data on laboratory, pharmacy, radiology, intensive care, inhalation therapy, room and board, and other charges were

Table 7.1: Mean Expenditures and Utilization Probabilities for Medical Care During the Last Year of Life (in 1980 dollars)

| | Month Prior to Death | | | | | | Inclusive | |
	6	5	4	3	2	1	Last 6 Months	Last Year[a]
All services								
Expenditures ($)	1,152	1,333	1,746	2,230	3,214	6,161	15,836	21,219
%[d]	100	100	100	100	100	100	100	100
p[c]	.69	.73	.78	.86	.88	1.00	1.00	1.00
Hospital inpatient								
Expenditures ($)	762	902	1,189	1,592	2,514	5,331	12,291	15,594
%	66	68	68	71	78	87	78	73
p	.25	.27	.35	.44	.56	.94	1.00	1.00
Physician[b]								
Expenditures ($)	281	317	394	437	501	616	2,546	3,942
%	24	24	23	20	16	10	16	19
p	.56	.59	.64	.71	.73	.88	.96	1.00

Hospital outpatient								
Expenditures ($)	76	67	98	116	87	52	498	964
%	7	5	6	5	3	1	3	5
p	.23	.26	.28	.31	.30	.24	.64	.79
Other[c]								
Expenditures ($)	33	46	64	85	112	161	501	719
%	3	3	4	4	3	3	3	3
p	.35	.40	.42	.45	.48	.48	.69	.76

Note: S. H. Long et al., "Medical Expenditures of Terminal Cancer Patients During the Last Year of Life," *Inquiry* 21 (Winter 1984): 318. Reprinted by permission of the publisher.

aBased on 662 cases for whom a full year of expenditure data were available.

bIncludes claims for physician services, other professional services, and other providers whose services are covered by Blue Shield Plans, such as medical equipment suppliers. Physician services account for more than 90 percent of the expenditures in this category.

cIncludes major medical and prescription drug claims as well as any Blue Cross Plan claims for nonhospital services such as home care and extended care facilities.

dPercent of expenditures for all services.

ePropability that medical services were used in each time period (based on claim records).

very stable over the six months prior to death. Even more pronounced than the pattern for total expenditures, hospital inpatient
expenses rise rapidly during the last two months of life. Fifty percent of hospital inpatient expenses for the last year of life occur
during the last two months, 34 percent in the last month alone.

This finding that hospital costs increase sharply in the last
two months of life for Blue Cross and Blue Shield members under
65 parallels findings about terminal costs in other populations. In
a study of deaths from all causes among the elderly, Lubitz and
Prihoda (1984) found that expenses in the last two months of life
comprised about 46 percent of all expenses in the last year. Two
studies on combined populations both under 65 and over 65 also
found that the expenditures increased as death approached.
Brooks and Smyth-Staruch (1984) found that in a nonhospice population in Ohio, 52 percent of all expenditures in the last 12 weeks
occurred in the final month. Spector and Mor (1984) found that 42
percent of all expenditures in the last six months of life were spent
in the last month.

The monthly probability of using physician services and the
associated charges also increased as death approached. Physician
services accounted for 19 percent of total expenditures in the last
year of life.

Expenditure Differences by Diagnosis and Demographic Characteristics

Of the differences in mean expenditures by diagnosis during the
last six months of life (data not shown), only those for hospital
inpatient care attained statistical significance at conventional levels after controlling for age, gender, state of residence, and com-
prehensiveness of insurance coverage. Hospital expenditures of
lung and colon-rectal cancer patients were somewhat higher than
those of breast cancer patients.[1]

There was little expenditure difference by age and sex. The
multivariate analysis revealed no significant differences in total
spending for all services or for hospital spending and utilization by
age group. Only the somewhat higher spending on physician care
by the youngest age group proved to be statistically significant.
The parameter estimate suggested that the terminal cancer
patients in the under 45 age group spent 36 percent ($p < .07$) more
for physician care than those in the 45 – 54 year cohort. After controlling for diagnosis, gender was not a significant determinant of

expenditure and utilization levels during the last six months of life.

Other studies have found age to be an important predictor of costs. Lubitz and Prihoda (1984) found a steady decline in average reimbursements per decedent as age increased in the Medicare population. In their analysis of the charges and utilization for 2,104 terminal cancer patients aged 21 and older, Spector and Mor (1984) found that six-month charges were inversely related to age. For each additional year of age, older cancer decedents accumulated $151 less in charges. The Spector and Mor study population included decedents both under and over age 65, and the age/cost relationship may be stronger in the elderly population if there is a tendency among providers to expend less effort and resources to prolong the lives of the "old" elderly than they do for the "younger" elderly.

Geographic Differences

The study found large geographic differences in expenditures. Table 7.2 displays the six-month expenditures and utilization for the three different state samples. Mean expenditures and inpatient days were considerably higher for the Michigan than the Indiana and Georgia cases.

A multivariate analysis was performed, using the cases from Michigan and Indiana, states that share a common border and are characterized by urban-rural diversity. (The Georgia sample was too small to include in this type of analysis.) Controlling for demographics, diagnoses and proportions of hospital, and physician and other services, the Michigan residents spent 63 percent more ($p < .0001$) than their Indiana counterparts on all services combined. Hospital and physician expenditures were estimated to be 68 percent ($p < .0001$) and 69 percent ($p < .001$) higher, respectively.

Some of the difference comes from the 20 percent greater ($p < .0001$) number of hospital days per Michigan patient, a gap too large to be explained by differences in the severity of cases among the several hundred observations in each state. This difference in days was unexpected, because hospital utilization for the general populations of the two states was nearly identical at the time of the study (no explanation for this finding is available). The rest of the difference in cost resulted from greater charges per day of inpatient care, despite similar patterns of room and ancillary services between the two samples. This remaining difference of over

Table 7.2: Mean Expenditures and Hospital Use for the Last Six Months of Life: Michigan, Indiana, and Georgia (Atlanta) (in 1980 dollars)

State	N	Hospital Total	Hospital Inpatient	Hospital Outpatient	Physician	Other	Hospital Admissions	Days
Michigan (percent of expenditures)	678	$18.666 (100%)	$14.590 (78%)	$687 (4%)	$2.966 (16%)	$423 (2%)	2.6	40.5
Indiana (percent of expenditures)	340	$10.752 (100%)	$8.106 (75%)	$124 (1%)	$1.817 (17%)	$704 (7%)	2.4	32.7
Georgia (Atlanta) (percent of expenditures)	36	$10.555 (100%)	$8.511 (81%)	$463 (4%)	$1.530 (14%)	$51 (1%)	3.0	32.1

40 percent in cost per day well exceeded total price differences alone.

For the Indiana sample, it was possible to compare costs for metropolitan and nonmetropolitan residents. Hospital expenses for metropolitan residents were 67 percent higher ($p < .01$), although physician spending did not vary significantly by metropolitan residence. The hospital difference was due primarily to the use of high-cost hospitals, since there was no significant difference in number of hospital days.

Discussion

The state variations in cost found in the Blue Cross and Blue Shield Association (BCBSA) study were due in part to utilization differences between samples that were presumably of similar illness severity. This suggests that there is potential for cost savings through utilization controls in the care of terminal cancer patients. Some cost reductions may come from changes in payment systems. Since the introduction of the Medicare prospective payment system, many Blue Cross and Blue Shield plans and other private payers have introduced new payment programs, often emphasizing per case rather than per diem reimbursement. Changes in payment incentives can cause significant changes in hospitalization patterns. Hospitals would have strong incentives to help find alternative care for the terminally ill if reimbursements were made at a fixed case rather than a per diem rate.

Per case reimbursement is also likely to be the most cost-effective way to reduce the cost of ancillary services. The BCBSA study found that the use of ancillary services remained fairly constant over the six-month period. Greater use of diagnostic testing and radiology treatment at the beginning of the six-month period, when curative medicine is probably still the goal, is understandable. The same level of diagnostic testing in the last two months is likely to be unnecessary, as well as intrusive and uncomfortable for the dying patient.

However, the greatest opportunity for cost reductions would result from reducing the use of the hospital in the last two months. The geographic differences in hospitalization rates in the last two months suggest that the decision to hospitalize may well be a result of "practice style," rather than medical necessity (Wennberg 1984). Hospice care, an increasingly available alternative to traditional terminal care, may be one way of reducing use of the hospital during the last one to two months of life.

COST CONTAINMENT AND
HOSPICE BENEFITS

In recent years, much attention has been focused on the cost-containment potential of hospice care. Insurance carriers and other third-party payers have included hospice care in group health benefit plans and publicly supported insurance programs. Most of the empirical research on the cost-effectiveness of hospice care has been associated with the Medicare age population (Spector and Mor 1984; Greer et al. 1986; Birmbaum and Kidder 1984; Hannan and O'Donnell 1984). In general, the results show that hospice care for terminally ill patients is less expensive to third-party payers than the cost of conventional care.

Published materials and data on the cost of terminal cancer care for a non-Medicare or younger population are relatively scarce. There is some indication that the cost of conventional care in the last stage of life is inversely related to the age of the patient. For each additional year of age, it was estimated that the cost of care would increase by $151 per patient. Largely because the costs of conventional care are greater in the younger population, hospice care appears to result in larger cost savings for non-Medicare patients (Spector and Mor 1984).

A project conducted by Blue Cross and Blue Shield of Massachusetts represents a systematic analysis of the potential cost savings of hospice care in the last six months of life (Narkiewicz 1986). The overall costs of hospice care were calculated from the first group of 95 terminal cancer patients who participated in the Massachusetts demonstration between 1981 and 1983. The mean age of the sample group was 54.4 years, with a range of 15 to 75 years of age. The Blue Cross and Blue Shield hospice benefit included a comprehensive package of medical and social services. Study results showed that the average length of stay was 54.4 days and the average total cost of hospice care was $11,051 per cancer patient. Table 7.3 shows a breakdown of costs by type of service. Hospital costs on average were $4,466, or 41 percent of total expenditures, while home care costs were $4,346 per patient, or 39 percent of total expenses. In contrast, hospital costs for conventional care averaged $12,291 or 78 percent of total expenditures in the last six months, while home care costs were less than 1 percent (Gibbs and Newman 1982).

The Massachusetts hospice population was compared to two control groups. Table 7.4 compares the costs of each of the last six months of life for the Massachusetts hospice patients and the pre-

Table 7.3:   Blue Cross and Blue Shield of Massachusetts'
Hospice Demonstration: Average Cost per Patient, Total and by
Service, 1981

Type of Service	Estimated Average Cost per Patient (N = 95)	Percent of Total Cost
Home care	$4,346	39%
Hospital inpatient	4,466	41
Skilled nursing facility	123	1
Extended benefits	284	2
Hospital outpatient department	768	7
Blue Shield physician services	1,964	10
Grand total	$11,051	100%

Note: Average length of stay for the 95 study patients was 54.4 days.

viously described BCBSA sample of terminally ill patients who
were covered by Blue Cross and Blue Shield of Michigan but did
not participate in a hospice program. Average charges for health
care services between the two states were standardized for
comparability.

The average expense per patient for hospice care was approximately $6,000 greater than nonhospice care over the total six-
month period. The average savings for hospice are evident in the
last month of life, when the cost of hospice was $6,457 per patient
and the expenditures for conventional care were $9,821 per
patient. Cost savings for hospice are not demonstrated in periods
prior to the last month of life. However, the savings per patient in
the last month are significantly large to offset relative losses in
other months. The financial gains associated with the hospice care
benefit in the last month of life are due to the substitution of home
care for expensive hospital days.

Table 7.4 shows that the hospice patients spent a compara-
tively greater number of hospital days over a six-month period.
Again, only in the last month of life did hospice care show a significant savings in hospital days and expenditures.

The Massachusetts demonstration also compared the hospice
sample group to a second control group that consisted of the prehospice experience of the 95 patients enrolled in the pilot hospice
program. Table 7.5 confirms that the greatest savings for hospice

Table 7.4: Average Costs per Patient in the Last Six Months of Life for Hospice and Conventional Care Patients, by Month Prior to Death, 1981–83

Month	Massachusetts Hospice (N = 95)			Michigan Conventional Care (N = 685)		
	Simple Average	Cumulative Average	Hospital Days	Simple Average	Cumulative Average	Hospital Days
1	$6.457	$6.457 (95)	9	$9.821	$9.821 (685)	16
2	6.659	13.116 (58)	9	4.726	14.547 (685)	9
3	4.966	18.082 (31)	8	3.133	17.680 (685)	6
4	5.349	23.431 (15)	10	2.223	19.903 (685)	4
5	3.375	26.806 (7)	8	1.731	21.634 (685)	3
6	2.443	29.249 (6)	5	1.534	23.168 (685)	3
Totals:	$29,249		49	$23,168		41

Notes: Total costs include hospital inpatient, hospital outpatient department, and home care services, and represent the average cost for patients who stayed in hospice from one month to six months. In addition, the numbers in parentheses represent the actual number of persons receiving hospice and conventional care benefits in each monthly period.

Table 7.5: Average Costs per Patient in the Last Six Months of Life for Massachusetts Hospice and Prehospice Groups, 1981

Month Prior to Death	Hospice Care		Prehospice Care	
	Simple Average	Cumulative	Simple Average	Cumulative
1	$6,457	$6,457 (95)	$9,918	$9,918[a]
2	6,659	13,116 (58)	5,504	15,422 (37)
3	4,966	18,082 (31)	5,144	20,506 (64)
4	5,349	23,431 (15)	3,453	24,019 (80)
5	3,375	26,806 (7)	2,567	26,586 (88)
6	2,443	29,249 (6)	1,847	28,433 (89)
Totals:	$29,249		$28,433	

Note: Numbers in parentheses represent the actual count of hospice and conventional care patients in the period.
[a]Represents adjusted costs reported in Michigan data, $N = 685$.

care occur in the last month of life, most likely because of substitution of hospice services for hospital days. Additional research is necessary to duplicate the above findings with a larger sample of patients in each time period prior to death. The small sample size of patients enrolled in hospice in months four, five, and six is indicative of the extent to which terminal cancer patients are involved in hospice early on in their illness.

Nonetheless, the results of the Massachusetts demonstration and other research on hospice care indicate that hospice care does not cost less than conventional care until the last month of life. One possible explanation for this common finding is that standard patterns of medical practice did not change for hospice patients, even though the philosophy of hospice care clearly discourages the use of curative medicine. Generally speaking, hospice programs offered to non-Medicare populations have had little control over the practice of conventional medicine for enrolled hospice patients, especially when they are hospitalized.

The hypothesis that patients enrolled in hospice programs are subject to conventional medicine receives some support from findings of the National Hospice Study (Greer et al. 1986). It was shown that both conventional patients and home-based hospice patients receive similar amounts of ancillary services upon admission to acute care hospitals. Apparently, home-based hospice programs lost control of their patients when they were admitted to the acute hospital. Another study on matched groups of children with terminal cancer showed that the costs of lab and other ancillary services were more than eightfold greater for patients who died in the hospital than for those who expired in the home (Moldow et al. 1982). At the home setting, medical ancillaries were provided or arranged by hospice program staff. This differential in cost is the result of medical practice patterns that may be performed without regard for medical appropriateness. Similarly, the Blue Cross and Blue Shield Association study mentioned earlier found that the ancillary cost of conventional care for terminal patients remained stable throughout the patient's last six months of life, even as death approached and diagnostic testing became irrelevant.

Studies on hospice programs clearly show that hospice care generates significantly lower costs in the last month of life relative to conventional care. The savings appear to be the result of a substitution of home care for hospital days, but they also result from the fact that a very large percentage of hospice patients enter the hospice only in the last month (Brooks and Smyth-Staruch 1984; Narkiewicz 1986). Studies have also found that hospice care is underutilized; about 10 percent of the terminally ill who are eligible for hospice actually enroll in this alternative (Brooks and Smyth-Staruch 1984). Increased use of hospice care in the last month of life offers third-party payers a significant opportunity for cost savings. There is potential for further savings if hospice programs achieve more control over medical care providers who continue to offer traditional curative treatment to patients who are enrolled in hospice programs. These hospice programs have no control over the delivery of patient services offered in hospitals and other traditional settings.

EXPENDITURES UNDER
COST-MANAGEMENT PROGRAMS

Employer interest in all forms of cost management remains very high. There has been only slight moderation in cost increases in recent years. Total expenditures on health care for the nation continues to show significant increases (*Medical Benefits* 1986). Many large employers are bracing for increases of 20 percent or more in traditional health insurance premium costs, primarily because of cost inflation (*Medical Benefits* 1987). A Wyatt Company survey of a representative sample of different-sized employers reveals that employers are adopting multiple cost-containment programs (The Wyatt Group 1986). Only 3 percent of the surveyed employers had not adopted any type of health care cost control. Cost-management efforts include a wide array of activities aimed at reducing or shifting costs. The most frequently chosen programs include cost sharing, second surgical opinion programs, benefit changes, preadmission review and other components of managed care, and alternative delivery systems such as health maintenance organizations and preferred provider organizations (PPOs).

In the last six years, most employers have amended their benefit plan designs to influence employee health care choices. Employers have redesigned benefits to include a wider range of alternatives to hospital care. According to the Wyatt Survey, only 7 percent of employers included home health care in their benefit packages in 1982, but by 1986, 75 percent had adopted it. In addition, 54 percent offered a separate hospice benefit in 1986. Another common change is an increase in cost sharing. The percentage of employers offering deductibles of over $100 in their benefit plans has increased from only 9 percent in 1982 to 55 percent in 1986, while the percentage with deductibles under $100 decreased from 40 percent to 3 percent.

The impact of increased cost sharing on the choices made by heavy users of health care services was examined in a survey by EQUICOR (1987). In this report, heavy use of health services was indicated if the patient was admitted to the hospital two or more times per year or stayed in the hospital more than 20 days per admission. Although the survey did not include terminal cancer patients, it is likely that they share the opinions and attitudes of respondents. Heavy users, the survey found, rarely considered price or out-of-pocket costs in their selection of doctors or hospitals. About 89 percent said they never considered price in their selection of doctors, while 20 percent said cost was not an important criterion in choosing a hospital. In contrast, 41 percent said the single most important criterion in choosing a hospital is a hospital's reputation for providing quality care. Thus, increased cost sharing is unlikely to change health care utilization of heavy users since cost is unimportant to them.

Another cost-containment strategy is to increase employee enrollment in HMOs. According to the Wyatt Survey, 63 percent of employers offered an HMO option in 1986. Among heavy users, only 9 percent were members of HMOs, but 35 percent of the non-HMO members were interested in joining HMOs. In theory, HMOs offer considerable potential for controlling the costs of terminal cancer care. HMOs are complete delivery systems that emphasize alternatives to hospital care. HMOs are more likely to control the use of hospital ancillaries when a terminal patient is hospitalized, because the HMO physician will follow the patient in all sites of care. HMOs also have financial incentives to provide the most cost-effective care. They manage costs through preadmission review and other managed care techniques, and they control access through the gatekeeper approach. As gatekeeper, a primary care physician must give prior approval to all specialty care.

Managed Care Programs

Another major effort to control the costs of private insurance has been the application of comprehensive managed care programs. Managed care usually includes preadmission review, concurrent review, second surgical opinion, discharge planning, and case management. Preadmission review or precertification of hospital stays requires the patient/employee or the physician/hospital to call a utilization review organization with information about the reasons for the proposed hospital admission, the treatment plan, and the estimated length of stay prior to admission. Registered nurse reviewers compare the information to established criteria in order to identify proposed hospitalizations that may be unnecessary and places where care may be rendered more cost effectively on an outpatient basis. When such potentially unnecessary hospitalizations are identified, the nurse reviewer refers the case to a physician consultant for a final decision. The review organization cannot deny any admissions but can advise the employer or insurance company that a particular admission was not medically necessary. Preadmission review programs have generated significant reductions in hospital care, depending upon the prior amount of unnecessary hospital use. Recent reports on the cost savings of preadmission review indicate that hospital admissions are reduced by 12.5 percent (Feldstein, Wickizer, and Wheeler 1988).

When a patient needs to stay longer than the initially requested and approved time, the physician/hospital must call the review organization to discuss the reasons for the increased length of stay. The utilization review program often tries to promote prompt discharge planning to facilitate earlier patient discharge from the hospital.

A relatively new addition to managed care programs is catastrophic case management. The objectives of catastrophic case management are to coordinate and organize the health care services needed by complicated cases in order to assure appropriate care, to maintain quality of care, and to provide the most cost-effective treatment possible. Case management programs will arrange for benefit coverage of appropriate alternative services not covered by the patient's insurance plan. A utilization review program may attempt to identify high-cost patients through clinical lists that target such conditions as spinal cord injury, high-risk neonates, respirator dependence, and AIDS. Terminal cancer patients may be identified through multiple admissions and high-cost admissions.

Preadmission review by itself may have little impact on reducing hospitalizations of terminal cancer patients in the last month of life. It is very unlikely that an employer would deny treatment at this point in the progress of the patient's condition. Preadmission review and concurrent review may be tools to distinguish terminal cancer patients from other cancer patients. In preadmission review, the nurse reviewer usually asks about the planned treatment or services in order to justify the admission. This identification is most likely to happen in the last month or two, when the potential for cost savings is greatest.

Once a terminal cancer case is identified, managed care programs may promote the most cost-effective setting for the patient's final care. If a hospice benefit is available, the preadmission review program would advise the physician of its availability and encourage its use. Case management services could provide highly individualized attention and appropriate alternatives to hospital care.

Blue Cross and Blue Shield of Colorado conducts a case management program for its Blue Cross and Blue Shield subscribers in metropolitan areas. Its method for identifying cases is unique and maximizes its potential for identifying terminal cancer patients. A nurse reviewer visits each hospital several times a week to review the medical record and meet with the hospital discharge planner as well as the attending physician to explore alternatives. If appropriate, an alternative care plan would be proposed to the patient and family. Although the case management program applies to all conditions, many terminal cancer patients have been identified and have participated in the program. Prior to 1987, Blue Cross and Blue Shield of Colorado did not offer a hospice benefit. Therefore, without the case management program, the alternative non-hospital care would not have been covered.

After identifying a case and the alternative treatment, the program administrator estimates the savings from reduced hospital days in advance of approving the benefit coverage extension. For example, one patient, a 60-year-old woman with metastatic cancer of the bladder, was hospitalized for 23 days prior to discharge to home hospice for seven days before expiring. In this case, seven days of hospital care were avoided, at a potential cost of $4,074, while the alternative care cost only $372 for net savings of $3,702. In another case, a 46-year-old woman with multiple sclerosis and metastatic cancer received 49 days of inpatient hospice care in lieu of 49 days of hospital care for a net savings of $12,235. Blue Cross and Blue Shield of Colorado saved over $60,000 on 12 terminal cancer patients in 1985 alone. Through this case management program, Blue Cross and Blue Shield of Colorado has proven to itself that hospice care can be cost effective and it has adopted a hospice benefit.

Case management programs have grown rapidly in the last three years. According to the Wyatt Survey, 18 percent of the surveyed employers now include case management as part of their health care cost-management programs. Appropriate case identification and timely intervention will remain key to increasing the impact of case management on the cost and quality of care for terminally ill cancer patients.

CONCLUSION

The costs of terminal cancer care are a significant part of the cost of health care for people under 65 as well as those over 65. The greatest proportion of the costs of terminal cancer care are for hospital care, especially in the last month of life. Within the limits of this data, the results show that cost savings exist in the last month of life. In addition, there are implications for further cost savings earlier on if hospice programs are able to maintain control over the medical practice patterns of traditional health care providers. Consequently, appropriate cost reductions may result from substituting expensive hospital care with less expensive alternatives such as home health care, home-based hospice, or appropriately controlled inpatient hospice. Some of the current health care cost-management strategies adopted by employers, such as cost sharing, will have little impact on reducing expenditures for terminal cancer patients. Through its highly individual approach, a catastrophic case management program offers significant potential for managing and reducing the costs of terminal care while promoting appropriate alternative care of good quality. The challenge in maximizing the cost-containment potential of case management is to identify terminal cancer patients through hospital preadmission review and prompt intervention. The success of this effort must await future evaluation.

NOTE

1. The multivariate estimates suggested that the hospital expenditures of lung and colon-rectal cancer patients are, respectively, 15 percent ($p < .10$) and 20 percent ($p < .05$) higher than those of breast cancer patients (Gibbs and Newman 1982).

REFERENCES

American Cancer Society. (1980). *Cancer Facts and Figures*. New York: American Cancer Society.

_____. (1981). *Cancer Facts and Figures*. New York: American Cancer Society.

Birmbaum, H. G., and Kidder, D. (1984). "What Does Hospice Cost?" *American Journal of Public Health* 74(7): 689 – 97.

Brooks, C. H., and Smyth-Staruch, K. (1984). "Hospice Home Care Cost Savings to Third-Party Insurers." *Medical Care* 22(8): 691.

EQUICOR. (1987). "EQUICOR Healthcare Survey—V. A Survey of Hospital Patients and Other Heavy Users of Healthcare Services." New York: EQUICOR (Equitable HCA Corporation).

Feldstein, P. J.; Wickizer, T. M.; and Wheeler, J. R. C. (1988). "The Effects of Utilization Review Programs on Health Care Use and Expenditures." *New England Journal of Medicine* 318(20): 1310 – 14.

Gibbs, J., and Newman, J. (1982). "Study of Health Services Used and Cost Incurred During the Last Six Months of a Terminal Illness." Final Report to U.S. Department of Health and Human Services. Chicago: Blue Cross and Blue Shield Association, Research and Development Department.

Greer, D.; Mor, V.; Morris, J.; Sheawood, S.; Kidder, D.; and Birmbaum, H. (1986). "An Alternative in Terminal Care: Results of the National Hospice Study." *Journal of Chronic Disease* 39(1): 9 – 26.

Hannan, E. L., and O'Donnell, J. F. (1984). "An Evaluation of Hospices in the New York State Hospice Demonstration Program." *Inquiry* 21(Winter): 338 – 48.

Lubitz, J., and Prihoda, R. (1984). "Use and Costs of Medicare Services in the Last Years of Life." In *Health United States 1983*. National Center for Health Statistics. DHHS Pub. No. (PHS) 84-1232. Washington, DC: U.S. Government Printing Office.

Medical Benefits. (1986). "U.S. Industrial Outlook, 1986: Health and Medical Services." *Medical Benefits: The Medical-Economic Digest*, 28 February.

_____. (1987). "Inflation Expected to Boost Indemnity Plan Rates." *Medical Benefits: The Medical-Economic Digest*, 31 January.

Moldow, D. G.; Armstrong, G.; Henry, W.; and Martinson, I. (1982). "The

Cost of Home Care for Dying Children." *Medical Care* 20(11): 1154 – 60.

Narkiewicz, R. D. (1986). "A Study of Hospice Costs for Non-Medicare Age Groups." *American Journal of Hospice Care* 3(1): 12 – 16.

National Center for Health Statistics. (1986). "Advance Report of Final Mortality Statistics, 1984." *Monthly Vital Statistics Report* 35(6), Supplement.

Spector, W., and Mor, V. (1984). "Utilization Charges for Terminal Cancer Patients in Rhode Island." *Inquiry* 21(Winter): 328 – 38.

Wennberg, J. (1984). "Dealing with Medical Practice Variations: A Proposal for Action." *Health Affairs* 3(2): 6 – 32.

The Wyatt Group. (1986). "1986 Group Benefits Survey: A Survey of Group Benefit Plans Covering Salaried Employees of U.S. Employers." Washington, DC: The Wyatt Company, Research and Information Center.

8 Site-Specific Treatment Costs for Cancer: An Analysis of the Medicare Continuous History Sample File

Mary S. Baker, Larry G. Kessler, and Robert C. Smucker

ABSTRACT.   The purpose of this analysis of the continuous Medicare history sample file was to derive information on the cost of treating cancers. The approach that was used for the analysis was to cumulate costs occurring during three postdiagnostic phases of the disease. The phases were defined in terms of treatment patterns: initial treatment (first three months following diagnosis), continuing care (interim between diagnosis and death), and terminal care (six months prior to death). Treatment phases were analyzed separately because medical expenses for cancer are significantly different during, for example, a first course of therapy and a period of surveillance for recurrence. Costs, expressed in 1984 dollars, were measured as cumulated charges made to Medicare for health care received during the specified time period of each cancer treatment phase. The site- and phase-specific costs reported here are intended to serve as raw materials for agencies and individuals interested in cost-effective planning of cancer-related health care activities.

Cancer is a disease that often requires medical attention in the form of treatment or surveillance over a long period of time. All cancer-associated costs that are accumulated during this period make up the incident or lifetime cost of treatment for the disease. It is this lifetime cost of treatment that could be eliminated or reduced by effective cancer control programs. The size of the potential savings in treatment costs attributable to cancer control cannot currently be estimated, however, because lifetime treatment costs have not been quantified. Some of the factors making quantification difficult include the following: a relatively unpredictable course of the disease; lack of suitable sources for cost information; presence of co-morbid conditions that may or may not be associated with the cancer; large variety of treatment options; rapidly changing medical technology; and variability of charges for services among different providers. Regardless of the difficulty, however, the scope of the cancer problem is such that costs cannot be ignored. About 5 million people alive today have at one time received a diagnosis of cancer (Feldman et al. 1986), and an estimated 965,000 new cases occurred in 1987 (American Cancer Society 1987). The growing extent of the cancer problem requires careful planning for future health care needs. This in turn requires accurate and up-to-date information on the cost of treatment. This study was initiated in order to meet those needs.

METHODS

Data Source

A copy of the continuous Medicare history sample file was obtained from the Office of Statistics and Data Administration, Health Care Financing Administration. The file is a 5 percent random sample of Medicare beneficiaries enrolled in 1974. It contains all Medicare activity from January 1, 1974 through December 31, 1981, for this cohort of 1.6 million beneficiaries. Data that are collected include inpatient hospital stays, skilled nursing facility stays, home health agency use, physician services, and outpatient care (Table 8.1). Medical expenditures that are not recorded in the CMHSF include prescribed medicines and nursing home care below the skilled level.

Table 8.1: Continuous Medicare History Sample File, 1974 – 81

A. Fixed Demographic Section
    1. Date of birth
    2. Date of death
    3. Sex
    4. Part A entitlement date
B. Inpatient Hospital Stay Section
    1. Date of admission
    2. Date of discharge
    3. Principle diagnosis
    4. Charges
C. Skilled Nursing Facility Stay Section
    1. Date of admission
    2. Date of discharge
    3. Diagnosis
    4. Charges
D. Home Health Agency Section
    1. Reference year
    2. Part A charges
    3. Part B charges
E. Outpatient Section
    1. Reference year
    2. Covered charges for outpatient services
    3. Covered charges for inpatient services
    4. Covered charges for other services
F. Payment Record Section
    1. Reference year
    2. Reasonable charges for non–hospital-based services
    3. Reasonable charges for physician services
    4. Reasonable charges for surgical services
    5. Reasonable charges for supplier services
    6. Reasonable charges for hospital services
    7. Psychiatric services

Note: Items from the continuous Medicare history sample file were used to construct an estimate of the total cost of treating each cancer site. Sections A – F are linked in the file through patient identifiers and claim numbers.

Plan for Analysis

The general plan for analysis of the file included the following steps: (1) create a subset of beneficiaries with cancer; (2) identify the date of cancer diagnosis for this subset; (3) use the date of diagnosis to assign costs recorded in the CMHSF to specific post-diagnostic time intervals. *Step 1*: Diagnoses may appear in two places in the CMHSF, at admission to an SNF and at discharge from a hospital. If either of these diagnoses were for cancer, the enrollee was placed in the cancer subset. *Step 2*: Since there is no indication in the CMHSF for "initial" cancer diagnosis, we defined it as the first cancer diagnosis to appear on a beneficiary's inpatient hospital record after a minimum of one year on the file without a cancer diagnosis. Enrollees whose initial diagnosis occurred in an SNF were excluded from the analysis because we believed they might contain a large proportion of cases not incident in the SNF. *Step 3*: Costs were assigned to postdiagnostic time intervals that were defined as follows: (1) initial treatment, first three months following diagnosis; (2) terminal treatment, final six months prior to death; (3) continuing care, interval between initial and terminal treatment.[1] For beneficiaries surviving less than nine months, costs were cumulated without subdivision into phases.

Provider "charges" rather than Medicare "reimbursements" were used to compute total treatment costs. The charges recorded in the CMHSF for hospitalization, stays in skilled nursing facilities, and home health services include deductibles and coinsurance amounts for stays or services that occur within the "benefit periods" defined by the Health Care Financing Administration. The definition of benefit period is adequate to cover most hospital and home health agency utilization. For SNF stays, however, a qualifying hospital stay is required prior to SNF admission in order for the stay to fall within a benefit period. If no qualifying stay occurs, charges for the SNF stay are registered as 0 in the CMHSF. Approximately 25 percent of SNF stays for persons in the cancer subset fall into this category. Since this represents a significant portion of medical expenses for cancer treatment, SNF charges were imputed where no prior qualifying stay had occurred. The imputation formula used was the length in days of nonqualified stay multiplied by the average daily SNF charge. Length of stay was computed from admission and discharge dates. In cases where no discharge date was given, the date of the end of the file, December 31, 1981, was used. The SNF average daily charge computed from qualified stays for the cancer subset was $73 in 1984 dollars.

The Medicare Supplementary Medical Insurance Plan (Part B) provides coverage for physicians' and other services, as well as outpatient hospital care. Part B charges do not include the annual deductible. For 1974–81, the annual deductible for Part B coverage was $60. Therefore, the sum of $60 was added to Part B charges for each beneficiary during years when expenses were incurred. For services listed under the Payment Record Section

(Table 8.1, F), Medicare pays approximately 80 percent (i.e., "reasonable charges"). Reasonable charges have been adjusted to reflect actual charges using the HCFA rate reduction factor for the years 1974 to 1981.

Assignment of Costs

The method of assignment of costs of disease phase differed for each section of the CMHSF as follows:

1. Inpatient Hospital Stay Section
    The date of hospital admission was used to assign hospital costs to initial, continuing, or terminal disease phases. The cost of the entire hospital stay was included in one phase only, regardless of date of discharge.

2. Skilled Nursing Facility Stay Section
    Both the admission date and date of discharge were used to assign SNF charges. Where SNF stays overlapped disease phase, costs were prorated based on the length of the stay occurring in each phase.

3. Home Health Agency (HHA) Section
    Charges for home health care are recorded in the CMHSF as yearly totals. Dates of provision of services are not recorded. Therefore, yearly totals were prorated to disease phases occurring within each year where HHA costs were reported.

4. Outpatient Section
    Outpatient charges are reported as yearly totals. They were treated similarly to HHA charges and prorated to disease phase.

5. Payment Record Section
    Charges in this section are reported as yearly totals. After adjusting "reasonable" charges to actual charges, costs were assigned to disease phase as for HHA and outpatient.

Charges associated with the initial and terminal phases were computed on a per patient basis and charges associated with the continuing care phase were computed on a per patient-month basis. Since charges for terminal care begin to appear about six months prior to death, the last six months of the file (July 1 – December 31, 1981) were not used for continuing care calculations, in order to avoid possible inclusion of terminal charges for cases who died just after the December 31, 1981 closing of the file. Persons receiving their initial diagnosis after April 1, 1981, with no valid death date, were excluded from the analysis because they could not be classified with respect to nine-month survival time.

Charges were assigned to specific cancer sites according to the ICD – 8 or ICD – 9 codes used in subsetting the CMHSF. Subsequent diagnoses that appear in hospital or SNF stay records were not considered for this analysis.

For comparative purposes, all dollar values (1974 – 81) in the CMHSF were adjusted to 1984 using the appropriate medical care component of the consumer price index (U.S. Department of Commerce 1985).

The standard error of the mean (SEM) was computed for all averaged charges so that calculation of confidence intervals is convenient for the reader.

RESULTS

Of the 1.6 million CMHSF enrollees, 125,832 qualified with an "initial" diagnosis of cancer. Thirteen diagnostic subcategories contained enough beneficiaries (> 1,000) to be analyzed. These are shown in Table 8.2 along with the numbers of beneficiaries in each group. Also shown is the number of beneficiaries in each group who survived less than nine months following initial diagnosis.

Phase-Specific Treatment Costs

Phase-specific treatment costs were computed for beneficiaries in each of the 13 cancer diagnostic groups. Results are shown in Table 8.3. Initial treatment was most expensive for beneficiaries with digestive system cancers, stomach ($14,443), colorectal ($14,190), and pancreatic ($14,009). Melanoma ($6,954) and breast ($7,606) were the least expensive. The difference in costs is probably due to the extent of surgery involved as well as the need for short-term post-surgical care.

Continuing care costs do not show as much variation by site as do initial treatment costs. Bladder ($766/month), lung ($690/month), and pancreatic cancers ($677/month) and all leukemias ($676/month) are relatively expensive while breast ($483/month) and uterine corpus cancers ($424/month) are less so. Continuing care expense is affected by the presence of co-morbid conditions. Also, use of the CMHSF may serve to bias continuing care toward an overestimate, since only the first seven

Table 8.2: Frequencies of CMHSF Enrollees with 13 Different Cancer Diagnoses

Initial Diagnosis	ICD-9 No.[a]	Frequencies		Total
		0-9 Month Survivors (percent of total)		
Colorectal	153-54	5,665	(28.8)	19,673
Lung	162	9,641	(62.7)	15,381
Prostate	185	2,743	(19.6)	14,002
Breast	174	1,724	(13.8)	12,486
Bladder	188	1,353	(19.8)	6,843
Leukemia	204-8	1,961	(52.4)	3,740
Pancreas	157	2,496	(77.3)	3,231
Stomach	151	1,889	(58.5)	3,228
Uterine corpus	182	432	(14.2)	3,042
Kidney	189	683	(35.0)	1,953
Ovary	183	740	(46.1)	1,605
Uterine cervix	180	311	(21.5)	1,448
Melanoma	172	196	(17.7)	1,105

[a]International Classifications of Diseases, 9th Revision, U.S. Department of Health and Human Services.

Table 8.3: Charges Made to Medicare for Treatment During the Initial, Continuing, and Terminal Phases of Cancer of 13 Sites (in 1984 dollars)

Cancer Site	Cancer Phase		Continuing (monthly)	Terminal (6 months)	
	Initial (3 months)				
Colorectal	$14,190	(96.5)[a]	$572	$15,776	(222.3)
Lung	12,916	(147.1)	690	15,565	(273.1)
Prostate	8,112	(69.4)	560	14,613	(283.2)
Breast	7,606	(58.1)	483	15,136	(301.9)
Bladder	8,470	(122.2)	766	18,577	(447.3)
Leukemia	9,068	(307.7)	676	19,777	(692.9)
Pancreas	14,009	(468.5)	677	14,790	(737.9)
Stomach	14,443	(314.7)	660	16,132	(639.5)
Uterine corpus	9,260	(134.8)	424	17,623	(741.2)
Kidney	12,608	(241.1)	670	19,302	(994.2)
Ovary	11,055	(272.5)	647	18,650	(867.9)
Uterine cervix	8,979	(269.6)	493	16,414	(924.6)
Melanoma	6,954	(201.8)	488	16,194	(905.9)
All sites combined	10,039	(35.1)	578	16,280	(98.7)

[a](Standard error of the mean)

Table 8.4: Charges Made to Medicare for 0−9 Month Survivors of Cancer of 13 Sites

Cancer Site	Total Charges	
Colorectal	$21,602	(245.2)[a]
Lung	17,957	(159.5)
Prostate	16,324	(272.3)
Breast	17,256	(380.1)
Bladder	22,670	(557.0)
Leukemia	18,929	(470.1)
Pancreas	17,876	(302.8)
Stomach	21,058	(455.1)
Uterine corpus	21,479	(866.9)
Kidney	21,861	(685.7)
Ovary	20,643	(638.8)
Uterine cervix	17,505	(900.9)
Melanoma	16,618	(1,021.5)
All sites combined	19,109	(81.5)

[a](Standard error of the mean)

years after diagnosis are available for analysis. These early years after diagnosis are more heavily monitored for recurrence and metastases in cancer patients than are the later years (Eiseman, Robinson, and Steele 1982). Thus, expenses should be greater. The cancers with high continuing care costs are primarily those with poor survival prognoses. Poor prognoses may lead to more intensive and expensive treatment.

Terminal care costs show the least variability by site when compared to the initial or continuing care phases of cancer treatment. For long-term survivors (Table 8.3), the terminal six months are most expensive for leukemia patients ($19,777) and least expensive for prostate cancer patients ($14,613). Still the difference is only 26 percent. Similarly, the total expenses for persons who survive less than nine months do not vary much by site (Table 8.4). Bladder cancer is high ($22,670) and prostate cancer is low ($16,324). The lack of variability in terminal costs may be a result of the palliative rather than curative nature of medical care. Palliative care is less likely to vary by site.

DISCUSSION

The CMHSF was used to derive estimates of the cost of treating cancers in the initial, continuing, and terminal phases of the disease. In subsequent research, these estimates can be used along with cancer incidence, survival, and mortality rates to compute population lifetime costs of treating cancers. Systematic, current, and comprehensive cost of treatment information for the general population has not been readily available. These findings should prove useful to persons and agencies responsible for allocating health care budgets and for planning cost-effective cancer treatment, screening, and prevention programs.

Limitations

The use of Medicare data to compute treatment costs has some drawbacks. Medicare coverage of medical expenses is not complete. In order to minimize the effect of limited coverage, we calculated and used charges made to Medicare by providers rather than reimbursements made by Medicare. The costs of nursing home care below the skilled level and prescribed medicines are omitted from this analysis, but together these two items have been estimated to represent less than 10 percent of cancer patients' treatment costs (Hodgson 1984). Although quality control analyses of CMHSF were not performed, HCFA performs consistency checks on all incoming claims. When inconsistencies are found, claims are returned to providers for corrections. In addition, HCFA statistical files are edited for inconsistencies. It is difficult to estimate quantitatively the reliability of data contained in the file. As an indication of reliability, however, we assessed the following inconsistencies: (1) frequencies of $0.00 or $1.00 charges for hospital stays, and (2) frequencies of the wrong sex indicator for sex-specific cancers. The cumulative percent of $0.00 and $1.00 charges for legitimate hospital stays, obviously erroneous charges, is 0.012 percent. The majority of charges (99.7 percent) are in the reasonable range of $101 – $50,000. Less conspicuous errors may be left uncorrected, however. The frequency of incorrect sex indicators that are recorded in the CMHSF is also very low. For example, 0.5 percent of beneficiaries diagnosed with cervical cancer are identified as males.

Although we expect that our estimates of costs are low due to the limitations of Medicare data, there are studies that indicate that the underestimate is not large. For example, in 1984 dollars, initial treatment for breast cancer at the Long Island Jewish Medical Center cost $10,345 (3,134 SEM) (Munoz et al. 1986). We report $7,606 (58 SEM). The cost of six months of terminal care for cancer patients in Rhode Island was reported as follows: lung,

$13,591; colorectal, $13,991; pancreas, $14,649; leukemia, $21,980; prostate, $12,068; and breast, $12,385; all adjusted to 1984 dollars (Spector and Mor 1984). These values are quite similar to those shown in Table 8.3. In some cases, the values are higher than those reported for Rhode Island, indicating that the bias in Medicare data is not severe and is not always toward the low end of the price range.

Implications

The costs of each phase by cancer site follow patterns that are expected from knowledge of the biological course of the disease and its clinical features and treatment. For example, cancers that are most expensive for the initial course of therapy—colorectal, pancreatic, and stomach cancer—involve extensive surgical procedures with sometimes lengthy recovery times. Cancers such as melanoma and breast cancer involve less intensive hospitalizations upon discovery of the malignancy and are also less expensive for initial therapy. These are the results that would be expected if the beneficiary's "initial" diagnosis had been correctly identified. Such consistencies with biological events lend support to the choice of analytical methodology.

Similarly, continuing care costs reflect degrees of clinical surveillance or complications. Bladder cancer is a site where routine testing (e.g., cystoscopies and cytologies) might well lead to higher continuing care costs, as shown in our results. Cancers of the female reproductive organs join melanoma and breast cancer as needing less costly monitoring during the continuing phase of the disease. However, taken together, monthly costs for the various cancer sites appear very high. It is important for the reader to remember several points made earlier. First, these "costs" reflect all charges to Medicare during the period between diagnosis and death, not just those attributable to cancer. The average charges per month for Medicare beneficiaries in a CMHSF subset generated randomly with regard to disease diagnosis were found to be $235. This represents a baseline from which to judge these continuing care costs for cancer. The population is an elderly one, with virtually no one under 65 years of age included here. But it should be clear that these figures reveal cancer to be an expensive disease among the elderly, even for those who survive the disease.

Terminal costs reflect charges accumulated during the last six months of life of those persons diagnosed with cancer, but not necessarily dying from cancer. Clinical care patterns recommended as conventional therapy, even in the terminal phase, are reflected in the cost patterns. For example, there is a limited degree of variability in terminal costs compared to initial and continuing care. This seems reasonable because, in the last stages of cancer, widespread metastases often cause functional failures that result in similar treatment patterns for diseases that began at different sites. The costs for those who died after a diagnosis of cancer were substantially higher than the average cost of death for the random subset patients, which was found to be approximately $11,000.

Direct medical expenses are only a portion of the cost of cancer. Indirect mortality and morbidity costs, as well as psychosocial costs, are equally devastating (Hodgson and Meiners 1982). It will be important to find a way of including these costs in the calculation of overall cancer costs on a large scale or routine basis. This report, covering direct medical costs only, represents a first step in the attempt to quantify the lifetime cost of treating cancer.

ACKNOWLEDGMENTS

The authors acknowledge Feather Davis, Gerald Riley, and Irving Goldstein at the Health Care Financing Administration for their assistance in obtaining and interpreting the Medicare data.

NOTE

1. The subdivision of cancer treatment into time intervals postdiagnosis was based on an examination of monthly hospital charges for beneficiaries having a cancer diagnosis. Charges were high for three months postdiagnosis, leveled off, then rose again approximately six months prior to death. Charges were not linearly distributed during initial and terminal phases.

REFERENCES

American Cancer Society. (1987). *Cancer Facts and Figures—1987*. New York: American Cancer Society.

Eiseman, B.; Robinson, W.; and Steele, G. (1982). *Follow-up of the Cancer Patient*. New York: Thieme-Stratton.

Feldman, A.; Kessler, L.; Myers, M.; and Naughton, D. (1986). "The prevalence of cancer." *New England Journal of Medicine* 315(22): 1394–97.

Hodgson, T. (1984). "The Economic Burden of Cancer." In *Proceedings of* the *Fourth National Conference of Human Values and Cancer*, 147 – 59. New York: American Cancer Society.

Hodgson, T., and Meiners, M. (1982). "Cost-of-Illness Methodology: A Guide to Current Practices and Procedures." *Milbank Memorial Fund Quarterly* 60:429 – 62.

Munoz, E.; Shamash, F.; Friedman, M.; Teicher, I.; and Wise, L. (1986). "Lumpectomy vs. Mastectomy." *Archives of Surgery* 121: 1297 – 1301.

Spector, W., and Mor, V. (1984). "Utilization and Charges for Terminal Cancer Patients in Rhode Island." *Inquiry* 21 (Winter): 328 – 37.

U.S. Department of Commerce. (1985). *Statistical Abstract of the United States 1986*. 106th Edition. Washington, DC: U.S. Government Printing Office.

9 The Changing Economic Burden of Cancer

Stuart O. Schweitzer

ABSTRACT.   The economic burden of cancer is dynamic, driven both by changing health care costs for cancer treatment and by changing patterns of cancer incidence. This chapter will use a variant of price index methodology to calculate the change in the economic burden of cancer that has occurred as a result of changing incidence of disease—both in the aggregate and by site. The issue is of interest because both the incidence and mortality rates have changed dramatically even in as short a period as the past decade. Changes by site of cancer have been both significant and uneven. These changes have resulted from a number of factors, including health behavior and medical technology. By analyzing the costs of cancer treatment by site, the author differentiates between those cancers in which significant gains can be achieved by cancer control measures, focused on prevention through changing health behaviors, and those in which gains cannot be achieved in this manner.

The economic burden of cancer is dynamic, driven by changing patterns of cancer incidence as well as changing costs of treatment. This chapter describes how a derivative of the consumer price index can be used to calculate the change in the economic burden of cancer that has occurred as a result of changing incidence of disease. The burden will be calculated for all cases of cancer taken together and also by site. The issue is of interest because both incidence and mortality rates of many types of cancer have changed dramatically even in as short a period as the past decade. These changes have resulted from a number of factors, including health behavior and medical technology. Changes in the burden of cancer by site have been both significant and uneven. By analyzing the burden of cancer by site, it is possible to differentiate between those cancers that are particularly amenable to cancer control measures, and those that are not.

BACKGROUND

Measuring the economic burden of disease recognizes that illness causes indirect as well as direct loss. While studies of the direct medical costs of treatment are numerous, analyses that include the broader burden that illness places on both patients and society are fewer in number. While direct costs pertain to costs of treatment of a disease, indirect costs attempt to measure the value of lost productivity caused by disability and premature death. Rice (1966) estimated the costs of nine disease categories. Her analysis measured the direct costs of hospital and nursing home care, physicians' and dentists' services, nursing care, and other professional services. In addition, the value of lost life and productivity was incorporated in the analysis. The indirect costs were found to be as great as the direct costs, thereby doubling the more common estimates of the cost of illness. This study was updated in 1976 (Cooper and Rice 1976) in a more comprehensive manner that included more disease categories as well as additional cost elements. More comprehensive and specific measures of the cost of illness enable more useful analyses of the allocation of scarce health services resources, for both the prevention and the treatment of illness.

This point is illustrated well in the controversy over policies concerning tobacco. Luce and Schweitzer (1978) estimated the total cost of illness produced by use of alcohol and tobacco. Subsequent studies updated and expanded these analyses (Leu and Schaub 1983; Warner 1984; Rice et al. 1986). Warner's work has been especially helpful in comparing alternative public policies toward control of smoking (Warner 1983, 1985, 1986).

The economic burden of disease is a function of two factors: the incidence of the disease and costs, both direct and indirect. The case of cancer is especially interesting to analyze because the pattern of disease within this broad category has changed so dramatically in recent years. Furthermore, the costs of treatment and the indirect costs of lost earnings vary widely by site. Age-adjusted incidence rates of uterine cancer, for example, fell between 15 and

30 percent between 1975 and 1985, while those of cancer of the lung and bronchus rose as much as 88 percent during this same period (U.S. Department of Health and Human Services 1988). Part of this change can be attributed to changing risk factors within the population, suggesting an important role for cancer control activities.

The implications of these varying trends in cancer incidence for the economic burden of cancer are that (1) the various types of cancer are treated differently, with different direct costs, and (2) the rates of disability and mortality that generate indirect costs differ as well. It is therefore useful to consider together changes in incidence rates, as well as total cost of disease, for the various sites of cancer.

METHODOLOGY

The approach used to determine the combined effect of incidence rates and costs is a variant of price index methodology. Two price index formulas are used in calculating changes in the overall cost of living, and for changes in costs within particular submarkets, such as medical care. Both use weights to adjust prices according to the importance of particular items in the "market basket" of goods and services. The Paasche index is calculated as follows:

$$I(P) = (\Sigma w_1 {}^* p_1)/(\Sigma w_1 {}^* p_0)$$

where the summations are made over all items, subscripts refer to time period—0 for baseline, and 1 for the later period—and w and p refer to weights and prices, respectively.

The Laspeyres index is calculated somewhat differently:

$$I(L) = (\Sigma w_0 {}^* p_1)/(\Sigma w_0 {}^* p_0)$$

The distinction between the two measures is that the Paasche index measures the ratio of expenditures required to purchase the current year's collection of commodities, while the Laspeyres index calculates the ratio of expenditures required to purchase the previous period's market basket. Both indices are similar in measuring the difference in expenditures required to purchase the same bundle of goods with different prices. Feldstein (1988) offers an excellent discussion of these two measures and the inadequacies of both. The Laspeyres index is used by the Bureau of Labor Statistics in computing the consumer price index and its components because it does not require recomputation of the market basket weights in each period.

One approach to measuring the changing burden of illness is to hold the costs of disease constant but allow the weights (incidence rates) of each cancer to vary. The formula for the Burden of Illness index (BI) is the following:

$$BI = (\Sigma w_1 {}^* p_0)/(\Sigma w_0 {}^* p_0)$$

with the same definitions of variables as used previously. The advantage of this version of the index, like the Laspeyres index, is that recomputation of price weights in each period, which is relatively difficult, is avoided. The incidence weights, on the other hand, are readily available from the National Cancer Institute from the Surveillance, Epidemiology, and End Results (SEER) program (U.S. Department of Health and Human Services 1988). Economic cost weights are obtained from Rice and Hodgson (1981). The definitions of disease categories are not exactly the same in the two sources, but they are nearly so.

RESULTS

Table 9.1 presents the age-adjusted incidence rates of cancer by site and by sex for whites and blacks for 1975 and 1985. The data illustrate substantial increases in the incidence rates for cancer of the lung and bronchus, prostate, and colon-rectum. Rates of stomach, uterine, and cervical cancer, however, have declined steeply.

The frequency of cancer cases by site for all sex/race groups in the two years is shown in Table 9.2. In both years, cancer of the lung and bronchus, colon/rectum, and breast are the most frequent, while cancers of the digestive system and of the female reproductive system are the least frequent.

These changing rates are multiplied by the total economic cost of illness as calculated by Rice. Two components of costs are used in the study: short stay hospital expense, and the indirect, lost earnings costs. Rice also presented ambulatory care costs in her 1981 study, but only for a limited number of cancer sites. Ambulatory care is a relatively small part of direct costs, ranging from 17 to 30 percent of the size of hospital care, but is under 10 percent of the total economic cost. We therefore omitted it from our analysis. Table 9.3 presents the 1975 total cancer costs by site, with the indirect costs calculated assuming a 6 percent discount rate applied to future lost earnings. Total costs are divided by the

Table 9.1: Age-Adjusted Cancer Incidence by Sex and Race, 1975 and 1985 (cases per million)

Site	White Male	Black Male	White Female	Black Female
1975				
Lung/bronchus	758	1,008	219	204
Colon/rectum	550	467	429	428
Oral cavity	181	173		
Stomach	125	198		
Esophagus	48	173		
Prostate	684	1,110		
Urinary bladder	286	136		
Breast			889	774
Corpus uteri			334	168
Ovary			144	100
Cervix			111	278
1985				
Lung/bronchus	805	1,247	352	384
Colon/rectum	623	569	450	435
Oral cavity	161	213		
Stomach	105	177		
Esophagus	52	184		
Prostate	834	1,255		
Urinary bladder	304	154		
Breast			1,042	877
Corpus uteri			231	142
Ovary			148	96
Cervix			74	152

Source: U.S. Department of Health and Human Services, 1988.

number of cases in 1975 to arrive at the per case costs, which are the weights used for both 1975 and 1985 incidence rates.

The aggregate cost of cancer, assuming constant per case costs, rose over 20 percent between 1975 and 1985, from $12.9 billion to $15.6 billion (Table 9.4). The change in cost was far from uniform, however, with some cancers increasing in cost, and others falling. The largest rates of increase are shown by cancer of the lung and bronchus and of the prostate. Each of these rose in cost by over 30 percent. Increases of over 20 percent occurred for colorectal, esophageal, and breast cancers. On the other hand, both cervical and uterine cancer costs declined nearly 30 percent during this period. Unfortunately, the absolute (rather than relative) declines in cervical and uterine cancer costs are small relative to the absolute rise in lung and bronchial cancer costs. In fact, nearly

Table 9.2: Cancer Cases and Distribution, 1975 and 1985

Site	Total Cases	Percent by Site
1975		
Lung/bronchus	104,220	20.6
Colon/rectum	101,906	20.2
Oral cavity	18,477	3.7
Stomach	13,679	2.7
Esophagus	6,387	1.3
Prostate	75,162	14.9
Urinary bladder	27,588	5.4
Breast	94,795	18.7
Corpus uteri	34,030	6.7
Ovary	15,027	3.0
Cervix	14,175	2.8
Total, all sites	505,446	100.0
1985		
Lung/bronchus	139,153	22.9
Colon/rectum	122,794	20.2
Oral cavity	18,857	3.1
Stomach	12,819	2.1
Esophagus	7,668	1.3
Prostate	99,759	16.4
Urinary bladder	32,205	5.3
Breast	121,490	20.0
Corpus uteri	26,136	4.3
Ovary	16,821	2.8
Cervix	9,991	1.6
Total, all sites	607,693	100.0

Source: U.S. Department of Health and Human Services, 1988.

one-third of the increase in the aggregate cost of cancer during this period is due to the increase in cost of cancer of the lung and bronchus. Lung and bronchus, oral cavity, and esophageal cancers, taken together, account for nearly one-half of the aggregate increase, with the other eight cancer sites making up the remaining half.

The right-hand column of Table 9.4 lists the distribution of aggregate cancer costs by site for each year. In each period, lung and bronchus cancer's share was more than double that of any other cancer site, accounting for approximately one-third of all cancer costs. Breast and colorectal cancers are also important in their share of total burden, with each accounting for approximately 15 percent of total costs. Esophageal cancer accounts for

Table 9.3: Direct and Indirect Costs for All Cancer Cases and
Cost per Case by Site, 1975

| Site | Total Costs ($ million) | | | Cost per Case ($) |
	Hospital	Indirect	Total	
Lung/bronchus	380	3,826	4,206	40,356
Colon/rectum	425	1,510	1,935	18,987
Oral cavity	67	408	475	25,707
Stomach	93	487	580	42,400
Esophagus	151	1,229	1,380	216,053
Prostate	169	402	571	7,596
Urinary bladder	178	522	700	25,373
Breast	344	1,537	1,881	19,842
Corpus uteri	78	163	241	7,081
Ovary	96	489	585	38,928
Cervix	124	327	451	31,815

Source: U.S. Department of Health and Human Services, 1988.

an additional 10 percent, while all of the others are relatively
small.

CONCLUSIONS

It is feasible to calculate the changing burden of illness by focusing
on changing patterns of disease, holding cost per case constant.
This merely turns the CPI on its side, for the CPI measures changing prices holding *quantities* constant. The Burden of Illness
index allows quantities to change, while holding *prices* constant.
While this is far from the whole story of the changing economic
burden of illness, it is an important one. One sees that in both
absolute and relative terms, the burden of cancer falls unevenly
across site. Potential savings are far greater in the more costly
types of cancer such as lung, colon, and breast. While savings
have been achieved for some cancers, most notably cervical and
uterine, they are less important in absolute terms than the others,
so those reduced costs have not done much to stem the rise of
aggregate cancer burden.

It is important to note that the cancer with the largest total
cost, cancer of the lung and bronchus, is also the site with the
largest percentage rise in total cost between 1975 and 1985. It is
also the cancer site that can be most effectively attacked by cancer
control measures, because its incidence is so closely related to
health behavior of the population. The success of life-style – based

Table 9.4: Total Costs and Distribution of Cancer by Site,
1975 and 1985

Site	1975 Total Cost ($ million)	Distribution by Site (%)
Lung/bronchus	4,206	32.7
Colon/rectum	1,935	15.0
Oral cavity	475	3.7
Stomach	580	4.6
Esophagus	1,380	10.7
Prostate	571	4.4
Urinary bladder	700	5.4
Breast	1,881	14.6
Corpus uteri	241	1.9
Ovary	585	4.5
Cervix	451	3.5
Total, all sites	12,876	100.0

Site	1985 Total Cost ($ million)	Distribution by Site (%)
Lung/bronchus	5,615	36.0
Colon/rectum	2,331	14.9
Oral cavity	484	3.1
Stomach	543	3.5
Esophagus	1,656	10.6
Prostate	757	4.8
Urinary bladder	666	4.3
Breast	2,410	15.4
Corpus uteri	185	1.2
Ovary	654	4.2
Cervix	317	2.0
Total, all sites	15,618	100.0

Source: U.S. Department of Health and Human Services, 1988.

health behavior programs is not universally positive, and yet successes have been achieved so that one can be encouraged that further gains are possible. Though much of the cancer cost story is bleak, the message for public policy is one of potential hope.

REFERENCES

Cooper, B. S., and Rice, D. P. (1976). "The Economic Cost of Illness Revisited." *Social Security Bulletin* 39(2): 21 – 36.

Feldstein, P. J. (1988). *Health Care Economics*. 3d ed. New York: Wiley & Sons.

Leu, R. E., and Schaub, T. (1983). "Does Smoking Increase Medical Care Expenditures?" *Social Science and Medicine* 17: 1907 – 14.

Luce, B., and Schweitzer, S. O. (1978). "Smoking and Alcohol Abuse: A Comparison of Their Economic Consequences." *The New England Journal of Medicine* 298(10): 569 – 71.

Rice, D. P. (1966). "Estimating the Cost of Illness." *Health Economics Series*, Series 6. Public Health Service. Washington, DC: U.S. Government Printing Office.

Rice, D. P., and Hodgson, T. A. (1981). "Social and Economic Implications of Cancer in the United States." National Center for Health Statistics. *Vital and Health Statistics*, Series 3, No. 20. DHHS Pub. No. (PHS) 81-1404. Washington, DC: U.S. Government Printing Office.

Rice, D. P.; Hodgson, T.; Sinsheimer, P.; Browner, W.; and Kopstein, A. (1986). "The Economic Costs of the Health Effects of Smoking, 1984." *The Milbank Quarterly* 64(4): 478 – 546.

U.S. Department of Health and Human Services. (1988). *Health United States 1987*. DHHS Pub. No. (PHS) 88-1232, p. 87. Washington, DC: U.S. Government Printing Office.

Warner, K. E. (1983). *The Benefits and Costs of Antismoking Policies*. Final Report. Grant No. HSO 3634. National Center for Health Services Research, OASH. Department of Health and Human Services. Washington, DC: U.S. Government Printing Office.

Warner, K. E. (1984). "The Economics of Smoking and Lung Cancer." In Loeb, L. A.; Ernster, V. L.; Warner, K. E.; Abbotts, J.; and Laszlo, J. "Smoking and Lung Cancer: An Overview." *Cancer Research* 44(12): 5940 – 58.

Warner, K. E. (1985). "Cigarette Advertising and Media Coverage of Smoking and Health." *The New England Journal of Medicine* 312(6): 384 – 88.

Warner, K. E. (1986). "Smoking and Health Implications of a Change in the Federal Cigarette Excise Tax." *Journal of the American Medical Association* 255(8): 1028 – 32.

Part IV

Perspectives on Cancer Care

The first three chapters in Part IV review the problems of diagnosis-related groups from the standpoints of the patient, the hospital, and the physician. Carol S. Viele describes two patients who have physical and emotional problems resulting from abbreviated hospital stays. She attributes the problems in these two cases to the DRG system, concluding that geriatric oncology patients have special needs that are not solved by the usual hospital utilization rules. Evidence shows that the DRG system of prospective reimbursement to hospitals has contributed to earlier hospital discharge. Hospital stays that are shorter than the assigned length of stay for a particular DRG are financially beneficial for the hospital, lengths of stay that are equivalent to the assigned days are financially neutral, and longer stays result in a financial burden to the hospital, if the patient is not found to be an outlier.

Charles H. White discusses the negative aspects of competition in the health field. He observes that the prospective payment system has reduced the number of admissions to hospitals, the average length of stay, and the volume of services and employees. He argues that another result has been a reduction in access to medical care, since insurance companies have instituted cost reduction rules and have increased patient copayments and deductibles.

Gary A. Ratkin states that patients are often denied the most appropriate treatment for cancer because third-party payers are reluctant to pay for protocol or experimental therapy. The fact that Medicare reimbursement for outpatient chemotherapy does not fully reimburse for the cost or administration of drugs has caused many oncologists to reconsider accepting these patients. He questions whether community hospitals and university medical centers can continue their involvement in clinical research without adequate reimbursement.

Viele, White, and Ratkin have underscored the problems for Medicare patients, hospitals, and oncologic care and research in these three chapters. Richard J. Steckel, the author of Chapter 13, also expresses concern about research funding, but from the viewpoint of the cancer center. Many cancer centers were established with funds from the National Cancer Institute and they continue to receive "core grants." These grants provide funds for support of the cancer center, for clinical research, and for patient care. A limited number of centers were exempted by HCFA from reimbursement through DRGs, and they continue to bill on a fee-for-service basis. Presumably, this will continue, although both the government and third-party payers state that they intend to restrict reimbursements to "service-related" costs. In that case, payment for research, for patient care during research protocol studies, and for professional training would diminish or vanish. Steckel urges that these and similar problems for cancer centers and academic centers should be carefully evaluated by the funding sources.

10 The Impact of DRGs on Geriatric Cancer Patients

Carol S. Viele

ABSTRACT. This chapter presents a description of diagnosis-related groups and the effect of the DRG system on two geriatric oncology patients. Both patients were admitted to a northern California university teaching hospital. The diagnosis, hospital course, and the effect of the DRG system on the duration and number of hospitalizations are described for each of these two patients. Also considered are the psychological and physical consequences of these experiences upon the two individuals.

When diagnosis-related groups were introduced in 1983, the medical and administrative communities assumed several different postures. One attitude was to ignore DRGs and hope that they would go away; another was to refuse to accept patients who were covered by Medicare. Both groups were aware of the reason for the development of DRGs; they were developed as a cost-control measure. Many persons were concerned that this new system of reimbursement would have an adverse effect upon their institutions.

Researchers at Yale University developed the DRG system, which is based upon the concept that patients can be classified into clinically meaningful groups. Patients within a given group are assumed to consume similar quantities of resources (e.g., tests, medications, nursing hours, and operating room time). The scheme is based upon the diagnosis established for the patient rather than upon the sophistication of the medical staff and of the hospital to which the patient is admitted. The DRGs are dependent on the patient's illness and treatment rather than upon a hospital's bed size, services provided, or the specialties of its medical staff (Grimaldi 1986, 6). This system, by its design, seems to penalize larger hospitals because of the availability (and support) of a large number of services and specialities that may be denied by the DRG system. It can also discriminate against patients who must seek care in smaller institutions where only limited services are offered.

Patients will normally be admitted to a hospital where their physician has privileges. Some patients are initially admitted to an institution that does not have the services they need (i.e., a neurosurgeon). The patient must then be moved to a center that has the services available. Depending upon the number of days the patient spent in the first institution, there may not be enough approved DRG days left for an adequate workup in the tertiary care center.

What are DRGs? They are subdivisions of 23 major diagnostic categories that represent the major body organs. A total of 467 DRGs are differentiated, defined, and assigned according to the following premises:

1. Principle diagnosis—the medical condition ultimately determined to have caused a hospitalization; the principal diagnosis may differ from the admitting diagnosis, which is a preliminary assessment of the reason for admission

2. Operating room (OR) procedure—a surgical procedure usually performed in an operating room

3. Complications or co-morbid condition (CC)—a secondary condition that arises during hospitalization or coexists at admission, and is thought to increase the length of stay by at least one day for about 75 percent of the patients

4. Age of the patient at admission—the three critical ages for DRG assignment are 17, 35, and 69 years of age

5. Patient's sex

6. Discharge status (i.e., dead or alive)

Of the variables listed above, only the principle diagnosis is used to assign each patient to a DRG. The other variables are used much less frequently (Grimaldi 1986, 6). The hospital medical record must be very explicit in detailing the reasons for hospitalization and for any compounding factors which may lengthen a patient's stay.

Before the introduction of DRGs, a patient could be admitted for one diagnosis and, while undergoing evaluation or treatment, have other serious problems recognized and treated. Under the DRG system, unrelated problems cannot be treated unless authorization is obtained. This ruling creates problems for many hospitalized patients, but especially for cancer patients. Patients must have a primary diagnosis, and any further workup must be justified and approved. The case studies that follow are just two examples of how the system has changed the concept of cancer care. Prior to DRGs, a patient with multiple symptoms would have a thorough search for the reasons for these problems. Those in the medical arena are now placed in the precarious position of being required to "treat and street" the patients as rapidly as possible.

As the cancer population ages, many problems become serious if left untreated. Under the DRG system, the patient is treated for one problem and others are left untreated. In addition, complications associated with the treatment may not be an acceptable reason for continued hospitalization. Although there is certainly a need for a cost-effective answer to this medical care dilemma, one wonders if the pendulum has swung too far away from meeting the patient's needs.

CASE STUDIES

How do the DRGs affect the patients with a diagnosis of cancer? The two cases discussed here are not meant to be all-inclusive, but they do illustrate some of the concerns of the hospital staff as they see what happens to patients under the DRG system.

The first case concerns Mrs. U., a 65-year-old woman who was found to have anaplastic thyroid carcinoma in 1985. A thyroidectomy was performed in 1985. She did well and was discharged four days after surgery. She resumed her normal activities and had no further difficulties until March of 1986. At that time, she was admitted with a two-week history of headache, loss of appetite, weakness, and paresthesias. Examination revealed a recurrent mass in her neck and metastases to the cervical spine. A neck exploration was performed and a diagnosis of recurrent cancer of the thyroid was established. A tracheostomy was done and a brace was applied to her neck because of instability of the cervical spine at C3 and C5.

Postoperatively, Mrs. U. had difficulty learning how to care for the tracheostomy. She was taught how to clean the tracheostomy cannula and to suction her trachea. The patient was hospitalized for 21 days for preoperative and postoperative care and initiation of chemotherapy of Cis-platinum, VP-16, and Prednisone for the recurrent cancer. Mrs. U. was given the usual premedication for nausea in an effort to prevent the nausea that usually accompanies Cis-platinum. She was to be discharged the day following therapy, according to the utilization review department. Because of severe nausea and inability to eat, she remained in the hospital for an additional 48 hours. She was decertified by the utilization review team and discharged. She was referred to a home care agency for continued training in the care of the tracheostomy.

Mrs. U. had been very independent prior to the second hospitalization. She was unmarried and lived alone. Her only relatives were two nieces. She was very frightened, had difficulty caring for herself, and did poorly with the self-care of the tracheostomy. She was trying, unsuccessfully, to cope with all the changes occurring in her body and her life-style.

Because she sustained a fall at home, she was seen in the emergency room and was readmitted to the hospital less than 24 hours after her discharge. Her blood chemistries showed a potassium level of 2.3 (normal value 3.0 – 5.5). Her niece related that she was unable to retain any food or fluids while she was at home. She was placed on intravenous feedings. Teaching was continued regarding tracheostomy care. She was hospitalized for four days during this admission and discharged to the care of a nursing agency. Under the Medicare regulations, nurses are only allowed a limited number of home visits. The number of visits is based upon the patient's needs for skilled nursing care. On discharge, the staff requested a daily visit for continued follow-up for tracheostomy teaching, but the patient was followed for only five days, based on the home care agency's assessment.

She was only home for two weeks when it became necessary to readmit her for an infection at the tracheostomy site with an organism called nafcillin-resistant staphylococcus aureus. The infection probably resulted from aspiration because she was not properly inflating the tracheostomy cuff while eating. She was hospitalized for ten days to receive intravenous antibiotics. Teaching regarding tracheostomy care was continued.

This discharge and readmission pattern continued for three months, during which she was hospitalized four times. During this time, her nieces learned to assist the patient with her tracheostomy and general care. A feeding gastrostomy was done to prevent aspiration pneumonia. Because of the Medicare DRG system and minimal length of stay allowed for her periods of hospitalization, she was never able to remain in the hospital long enough to truly stabilize her disease. Because of this patient's inability to learn to care for her tracheostomy, infections were the major obstacle to further administration of chemotherapy. Radiation was not an option, due to the infection of her neck wound and possible inhibition of healing.

This case presents an example of the problems the DRG system can cause for an individual who has had to live within the reimbursement system and deal with its inadequacies. The system is not designed for the individual. It was established to treat all individuals with similar diagnoses alike and, since no two persons are the same, many problems arise. This patient had a number of admissions to the hospital that were not reimbursed. She was never judged to be too ill to warrant continued hospitalization from a medical standpoint. The problem was really a social one, since neither she nor her family could provide the nursing care she needed.

The second case, Mr. D., is a 68-year-old male patient who was admitted with a diagnosis of multiple myeloma and pneumocystis pneumonia (PCP). Mr. D. had been dealing successfully with the diagnosis and treatment of multiple myeloma for five years. His myeloma was asymptomatic. Eventually, however, he developed a dry cough accompanied by shortness of breath. His wife of 35 years became very concerned about his condition when he began to run a fever.

He came to the hospital after his fever reached 102°F for two consecutive days. It was very difficult for him to comprehend the additional diagnosis of pneumocystis pneumonia. This anxiety was increased by his knowledge that pneumocystis pneumonia can be related to acquired immune deficiency syndrome (AIDS). It was necessary to deal with Mr. D. on both a physical and psychological level. He was treated with intravenous antibiotics (Septa) for seven days, then switched to the oral form of the medication and sent home to continue a two-week course of antibiotics. Before the end of two weeks, he suffered a grand mal seizure and was brought to the emergency room by ambulance on Friday evening. When Mr. D. had stabilized, Mrs. D. asked if he should have been discharged so soon. The patient had a thorough neurological examination by a neurologist. He also had a lumbar puncture, computerized tomography (CT) scan, and an electroencephalogram (EEG), all of which were within normal limits. No reason for his seizure could be found. On the third day of hospitalization, he was told that all further workup would be done as an outpatient, due to the restrictions of DRGs. He and his wife were very concerned about discharge so soon after his seizure. He was told that if any further problems developed he should return to the hospital immediately.

These two cases demonstrate that the DRG system has major limitations for Medicare cancer patients. It is an accepted fact that medical care must be provided in a cost-effective manner, but something is missing when patients are rehospitalized with this degree of frequency. Both the patients and their families perceived that they were discharged hastily, and that the reasons for early discharge were dictated by DRGs. The medical system should keep patients in the hospital until their treatment is complete or until discharge will not adversely affect their illness. Patients have a right to expect a level of care that provides the length of hospitalization needed for recovery from the illness that initially brought them to the hospital.

These cases demonstrate that this degree of care was not adequately met. Medical professionals must provide better quality care to this needy population. The geriatric oncology patient has very special needs, which must be fulfilled in a conscientious, cost-effective, and high-quality manner. With the awareness of situations such as those described above, perhaps the medical profession can attempt to influence legislation to provide for the high-quality care that cancer patients and all sick patients deserve.

CONCLUSION

In conclusion, the words of John F. Kennedy serve as a reminder of the ideals that should guide our assessment of the DRG system: "For of those to whom much is given, much is required. And when at some future date the high court of history sits in judgement on each of us, recording whether in our brief span of service we fulfilled our responsibilities to the state, our success or failure, in whatever office we hold, will be measured by the answers to four questions: First, were we truly men of courage . . . Second, were we truly men of judgement . . . Third, were we truly men of integrity . . . Finally, were we truly men of dedication?" (Kennedy 1961).

REFERENCES

Grimaldi, P. L. (1986). "DRGs and Long Term Care." *American Health Care Association Journal*, January: 6 – 9.

Kennedy, J. F. (1961). Speech to the Massachusetts State Legislature. Boston, January 9.

SELECTED BIBLIOGRAPHY

Adams, R., and Johnson, B. "Acuity and Staffing Under Prospective Payment." *Journal of Nursing Administration* 16, no. 10 (October 1986): 21 – 25.

Grimaldi, P. L. "DRGs and Long Term Care." *American Health Care Association Journal* (January 1986): 6 – 9.

Harron, J., and Schaeffer, J. "DRGs and the Intensity of Skilled Nursing." *Geriatric Nursing* (January – February 1986): 31 – 33.

Horn, S. D.; Sharkey, P. D.; Chambers, A. F.; and Horn, R. D. "Severity of Illness Within DRGs: Impact on Prospective Payment." *American Journal of Public Health* 75, no. 10 (1985): 39 – 40.

Jenkins, L. "A Perfect Match?" *Nursing Times* March 19, 1986, 39 – 40.

McCormick, B. "What's the Cost of Nursing Care?" *Hospitals* 60, no. 21 (1986): 46 – 52.

McKibbin, R.; Brimmer, P.; Galliher, J.; Hartley, S.; and Clinton, J. "Nursing Costs and DRG Payments." *American Journal of Nursing* 85, no. 12 (1985): 1353 – 56.

Mundinger, M. "DRGs: A Glass Half Full for Nursing." *Nursing Outlook* (November – December 1985): 265.

Prescott, P. "DRG Prospective Reimbursement: The Nursing Intensity Factor." *Nursing Management* 17, no. 1 (1986): 43 – 46.

Sherman, J. "DRG 001: A Multihospital Comparison." *Nursing Management* 17, no. 10 (1986): 17 – 20.

Smeltzer, C., and Flores, S. "DRGs: What Nurses Need to Know." *Nursing Management* 17, no. 10 (1986): 43 – 48.

Taylor, M. "The Effect of DRGs on Home Health Care." *Nursing Outlook* 33, no. 6 (1985): 288 – 89.

Thomas, S., and Wood, T. "Nursing and the DRG System." *The Australian Nurses Journal* 15, no. 4 (1985): 50 – 52.

11 Cost and Quality: The Hospital Perspective

Charles H. White

ABSTRACT. Hospitals are searching for a balance between cost and quality in the new era of price-sensitive competition. Different financial incentives have had an impact on patients, medical practice, and hospital financial viability. This chapter explores the political and economic assumptions underlying payment systems intended to reduce overutilization of hospital inpatient care and contain continued growth of costs. The competitive marketplace in health care has achieved many of its goals and has encouraged changes in the behavior of the public as well as providers. Special attention is devoted to the unique interests of cancer care and the various parties that are interested in that care.

Hospitals are searching for a balance between cost and quality. They are searching for the right balance between their mission of providing responsible care and their need to conserve resources. Only by finding this balance will they continue to exist.

COST AND QUALITY

Both words—"cost" and "quality"—have many connotations. To government personnel, "cost" refers to the appropriation in the governor's or president's budget. Blue Cross sees cost as how many claims are being paid. To a hospital, cost of care is a simple subtraction problem: subtract cost from payment. Today, however, one more often subtracts payment from cost for delivering inpatient care, which can result in a negative balance. The reason, of course, is that Medi-Cal hospital contracts, Medicare diagnosis-related groups, and negotiated third-party payer contracts have fixed or "capped" payments that may be unrelated to the actual costs of delivering care. In 1988, more than half of California's hospitals expected to lose money on inpatient services (California Association of Hospitals and Health Systems 1988a).

The largest allocation of funding for research, treatment, and prevention by the U.S. Congress over the past 30 years went to heart disease, followed by cancer, then stroke. These federal expenditures represent the level of emphasis given to each disease as a matter of public policy. Obviously, cancer is of concern to the government and to the public. And that concern justifies an evaluation of the effect of the new DRG payment system upon the cancer patient.

The government and health care insurers have developed a health care system that establishes competition between health care providers. In this marketplace system, price-sensitive negotiations are conducted between payers and the providers of patient care. This chapter will discuss the impact of this competitive economic system on health care delivery.

Competition in health care was created with the erroneous belief at the governmental level that there was a great amount of waste in the health care system and that, if the waste could be eliminated, costs would go down. Equally erroneous was the assumption that competition would reduce quality of care.

A more accurate assumption was that primary care gatekeeper physicians, along with strict utilization review and tighter claims administration, would reduce costs to payers by restricting the supply of care. Equally accurate was the assumption that increasing out-of-pocket costs to patients and families would reduce the demand for care.

The competitive system had the immediate effect of reducing the following characteristics of hospitals: number of admissions, length of patient stay, volume of surgery, diagnostic tests, x-rays, ancillary services (DRGs do regulate the use of ancillary services), nursing hours, intensive care, total hospital employment, and nurse employment (White and Morse 1985; White and Lewis 1986). Cash flow was also reduced, particularly for small and rural hospitals. Another noticeable change in practice in hospital inpatient care can be seen in the reduction of standing orders for preadmission testing and prior day admissions. These services were considered to be routine by most hospitals, although additional costs were generated. The physician was assisted in gaining information while the patient gained some comfort and convenience. In a price-sensitive marketplace, under the pressure of limited payment systems, these familiar routines were discontinued almost overnight because payers denied approval.

Other Consequences of Competition

Other changes have occurred in medical practice as a result of the competitive system. Access to care has changed for many people as third-party payers attempt to reduce costs. Hospital emergency rooms have become the point of entry to the health care system for those unable to afford private medical care. Simultaneously, patient copayments and deductibles have increased.

Accounts receivable have increased in many hospitals. Furthermore, the turnover time on accounts receivable has risen from 30 to 70 days on the average in California hospitals. Research shows that turnover time on Medi-Cal accounts receivable is up to 150 days (White and Morse 1985), and some estimates are even higher. Waiting longer to be paid less for giving more service is another product of the competitive system.

Empty beds, accompanied by rising levels of acuity or severity of illness, are also consequences of competition. Any nurse will agree that inpatients are sicker, that severity levels of illness are rising.

Payers believe that their salvation for reducing costs lies in shifting financial risk and cost to other health care settings, particularly outpatient. Again, anyone who works in one of those ambulatory settings will agree that the average level of acuity is rising.

Effects on Medical Practice

It is possible to draw some conclusions about the results of a health care marketplace. Competitive, price-sensitive health care has produced the truism, "Practice follows payment." It has come as a great shock to some that the practice of medicine does not always follow those patterns taught in medical school. In the hospital world of today, however, health care is directed to that level of care for which somebody is willing to pay. Many surgical procedures are reimbursed only if performed in an outpatient setting. Many hospital admissions are denied, unless the need for acute care can be documented.

Biomedical ethics issues and increased uncompensated care are other indicators of the competitive environment. Decisions about allocations of resources and choices to withhold or withdraw treatment are increasingly confronted in the courts.

The phrase "no care zone" is wonderfully apt for pointing out that there are large gaps in our health care system that prevent continuity of care and inhibit access for some of our citizens. Reduced funding decreases the ability of providers to furnish charity or no-pay care.

SHIFT OF COST AND RISK

The competitive system was intended to shift costs and financial risk in the delivery of care. In the Medi-Cal selective contracting program, the shift of financial risk was to hospitals; in the Medicare prospective payment system, risks were shifted to hospitals and additional costs to patients; and for insurers and employers the shift was to hospitals, physicians, and patients through increased use of copayments, deductibles, fee schedules, and negotiated flat rate contracts. The end result has been an uneasy political balance achieved by reducing both the supply of care (by doctors and hospitals) and the demand for care (by patients and families).

On the other hand, competitive incentives developed by the private payer systems have achieved more cost savings and changes in patterns of health care delivery than previous attempts by regulatory approaches. Hospital cost-containment programs in several states have been discontinued as ineffective because only hospital incentives were controlled, not physicians or patients.

Professional Review Organizations as Sentinels

One of the federal government's basic assumptions underlying the creation of the prospective payment system was that a large number of Medicare patients would be readmitted to hospitals. In other words, since doctors and hospitals would play games to try to get around the system and maximize payments, a sentinel—the professional review organization (PRO)—would be needed. However, less than 2 percent of the expected numbers of readmissions actually occurred (White 1986b). Quality of care problems did not materialize either. Fewer than 10 percent of the expected numbers of anticipated problem cases have been located by the PROs (White 1986b). The PROs were created on the false assumption that doctors were giving bad care and that hospitals were wasteful. As the DRG rates have been phased in, the results have been transfer of care to other settings, lower utilization, and few admissions. Those effects were predicted and, indeed, desired by the sponsors of prospective payment. Hospitals have been accused of profit making, even though nearly half of all California facilities are losing money (California Association of Hospitals and Health Systems 1988b). We must remember that the early years (1983 – 87) of prospective payment and competition were also a time of lower rates of inflation; otherwise, financial losses might have been worse.

Still, competition does work. It works well for some patients, some hospitals, some doctors, and most of the payers. The competition system does benefit some people, but they may not be the same people for whom the American Cancer Society and other health care professionals are the major advocates.

Of course, the health care marketplace is still relatively new, and we have not yet achieved the national level of Medicare reimbursement that will provide approximately the same level of DRG payments to each hospital. The ultimate objective of moving toward a national level is that Mississippi hospitals will receive as much reimbursement as those in San Francisco after appropriate labor adjustments, disregarding hospital, patient, or physician characteristics. The hospital industry is sorely divided on this issue, and its lack of consensus has been a political weakness.

Effects on Types of Hospitals

The era of cost reimbursement enabled investor-owned hospitals to grow and succeed. Despite all the rhetoric, corporate hospitals had one prime characteristic that was neither staffing nor better management. Investor-owned hospitals performed more ancillary services per patient-day than nonprofit or government-owned hospitals. More surgeries, more x-rays, more tests—more ancillary services of all types. Each of these was reimbursed separately on a fee-for-service basis, with cost reimbursement able to pay the bills. Profit margins were built upon this foundation of ancillary services.

The competitive system, by contrast, led to increasing growth of HMOs and PPOs in the belief that a primary gatekeeper system would save money by reducing specialty care and hospital admissions, and the use of ancillary services. If the fee-for-service, cost-based system encouraged overutilization, then the prominent features now in existence—DRG payments, Medi-Cal per diem contracts, and negotiated rates with payers—are incentives for underutilization. Underutilization incentives and restrictions have created serious financial problems for the investor-owned hospital industry.

Nonprofit community hospitals succeeded as independent facilities in the era before DRGs and prospective payment. Public hospitals were paid more than half of their charges and could continue to provide uncompensated care to public patients by cost shifting from private patients, along with tax revenue support.

It has become clear that competition favors HMOs by encouraging less inpatient utilization, more outpatient care, and more preventive medicine. Thus, HMO organizations are growing all over the United States, particularly in the large urban areas in the East, where groups of patients can be added.

The competitive system is destroying the public hospitals by replacing paying patients with nonpaying patients. Competition breeds uncompensated care, and this is the political issue that will change the system. The present approach to competition is an interim. It is temporary. Health care in the United States is on its way to another form of practice and payment. Uncompensated care will be the straw that breaks the back of the system.

IMPACT ON THE PUBLIC

Perhaps the most startling conclusion drawn from studies is that there is no discernible difference in quality brought about by the competitive marketplace (White 1986b). There have been no documented examples of patient care decisions made by physicians or nurses based upon cost considerations, despite predictions of lowered quality and accusations of "sicker but quicker" premature discharges.

The public has responded to competition far more than government or the insurers had expected. Wellness has gained credibility, people have changed diets and life-styles, and they are willing to pay copayments and deductibles. Many suppositions about individual responsibility for health have changed, probably for the better. Many more patients are sharing in decisions about their care with their physicians.

DRG AVERAGES

The DRG prospective payment system is based on the theory of averaging. It was assumed that there would be some expensive cases (outliers) and that all of the rest of the cases (inliers) would balance the economic effect of outliers so that hospitals would break even. In theory, profit from the inliers would balance losses from the outliers. An outlier could be an extra long stay (day outlier), or a high-acuity, more complex case (cost outlier). Thus, if a hospital could discharge a patient one or more days before the end of the average length of stay for that DRG, or did not need to supply as many services as the DRG allowed, the excess money could be retained. Prospective payment thus created a profit margin financial incentive that, in theory, would help keep the hospital solvent.

However, like most federal assumptions, the averaging theory has not proved true. The national average shows that about 6 percent of all Medicare patients are outliers (White 1986a). If a hospital shows a large number of outliers, or has a large number of high-severity patients, the result will be financial losses from inadequate Medicare DRG payment. The 6 percent outlier tail could, therefore, wag the 94 percent dog of inpatient care, resulting in a new loss from Medicare inpatient services for those hospitals with an unusual number of complex cases.

Cancer-related issues do not appear to be a major part of the outliers that are creating large dollar losses. Very few outliers appear from surgical cases; some of the loss is in internal medicine, but most is in pulmonary cases, probably related to flu epidemics. Nevertheless, outliers are becoming a great burden to many hospitals, and the Medicare program must adjust reimbursement for them. An upward adjustment was indeed proposed for the federal budget for 1989.

IMPACT ON ONCOLOGY UNITS

Reductions in federal funding for health research and services will surely affect the programs of medical schools and teaching hospitals. In community hospitals, this loss of funding will prevent the medical staff from participating in protocol studies and clinical trials. Lack of net revenue margins for community hospitals could also result in slower diffusion of new medical technology. A definite reduction in the provision of the latest advances in cancer care would result.

Hospital-based oncology units are very rich in staffing mix in order to provide appropriate services to cancer patients. A higher than average number of full-time equivalents (FTEs), resulting in higher than average salary and wage expenditures for the oncology unit, might point out a target when budget reductions are necessary. So far, however, we have seen no evidence that facilities have reduced the mixture of well-trained staff in oncology in order to save money.

The good news is that, because of their dedication, hospital medical staff spend a great deal of time working hard to restrain expenses—to their everlasting credit. They have refocused their efforts to control costs, but all the evidence suggests that their first concern is still quality. Doctors and hospitals are firmly focused on whatever effort is necessary to deliver high-quality care. Quality comes before cost.

The last feature of competition is the advent of marketing and advertising. The only health occupation in hospital employment that increased during calendar year 1986 was planning and marketing. One of the truisms of marketing in hospitals is that specific units must be advertised—a cancer center, a weight loss program, sports medicine, or any other. This is a kind of "boutique approach." In retail marketing, Macy's stores have demonstrated success at this technique and have dominated their competition by developing specialty centers. This "centers of excellence" approach in hospital marketing will produce a better overall public perception of quality. Advertising agencies insist that when a public opinion poll asks the question, "What's the best hospital in your area?," people will answer with the name of the hospital that advertises individual special care units. In this case, the overall perception of quality is more than the sum of its individual parts.

Hospital-based services or free-standing centers that offer comprehensive cancer care seem well adapted to the competitive environment. It is important that hospitals and medical staff pay strict attention to high quality, that they control costs and inappropriate utilization, advertise and market their best strengths, and keep searching for the right balance.

SUMMARY

The competitive marketplace in health care has earned a mixed score, exhibiting both strengths and weaknesses. Governmental bodies at state and federal levels have discovered that it is possible to change the health care delivery system; it is possible to reduce spending by adjusting financial incentives for patients and providers.

Perhaps the most encouraging outcome of the competitive marketplace is that the American public has responded to new options and choices of health plans. In addition, new patterns of care can still boast of very high quality. On the other hand, growth of uncompensated care and strains on rural hospitals remind us that no payment system yet implemented has been without flaws, and that many systems amount to an exchange of one set of problems for another.

The health care delivery system is now thoroughly enmeshed in the political process; it will shrink or expand along with the economy and as public policy decisions change with each new leader. The next federal administration will have its hand in determining what will follow this competitive era in health care.

REFERENCES

California Association of Hospitals and Health Systems (1988a). "Editorial." *California Hospitals* (June): 5

_____. (1988b). "Health Care Issues in California." Congressional Briefing Document, June: vii.

White, C. H. (1986a). "Competition Incentives: Smaller Carrot, Bigger Stick." *Western Journal of Medicine* 145(4): 535 – 36.

_____. (1986b). "Evaluation of the California Professional Review Organization: The First Two Years, 1983 – 85." Paper prepared for the Joint PRO Evaluation Task Force. California Medical Association/California Hospital Association, May.

White, C. H., and Lewis, S. (1986). *Strategic Planning Assumptions for Hospitals 1987 – 89*. Sacramento, CA: California Hospital Association.

White, C. H., and Morse, L. H. (1985). *Hospital Fact Book*. Sacramento, CA: California Hospital Association.

12 A Professional Perspective on the Issue

Gary A. Ratkin

ABSTRACT. Cost containment poses many economic problems to the oncologist. Prospective payment systems underestimate the severity of illness or the complexity of care for cancer diagnosis-related groups. Reimbursement for outpatient cancer treatments is inadequate and discourages physicians from accepting assignments or treating Medicare patients. Clinical research in oncology is negatively affected by cost-containment efforts that limit hospital stays or limit payment for investigational therapy. Managed health care programs (HMOs) provide economic incentives to limit the use of new technologies or referral to cancer specialists. In this chapter, suggestions are made to provide data on the cost of oncology care so that adequate reimbursement for humane, cost-effective treatment for cancer patients can be implemented.

Medical oncologists fulfill a number of roles in carrying out their daily responsibilities. The oncologist may act as a consultant on cancer diagnosis, as a practitioner in workup and management, as a provider of chemotherapy, as a clinical investigator, and as an educator to other health care professionals and the public. Today, each of these roles must be conducted under the umbrella of cost control.

Cancer evaluation and treatment is rapidly changing with new diagnostic techniques, treatment modalities, and specialists becoming widely available. The *Wall Street Journal* (24 April 1987) reported on a new type of consumer advocate-consultant who directs patients through the confusing maze of cancer resources, subspecialists, and treatment regimens now available to patients. It is rare for a cancer patient today to have one physician manage all the aspects of his or her care.

This chapter describes the difficulties our physicians and practices face in delivering modern care in this era of strict cost containment. While oncologists deal with prospective payment systems, managed health care programs, and increased demand for outpatient services, we must also speak out for quality care and patient access to adequate specialty referrals.

THE IMPACT OF PROSPECTIVE PAYMENT SYSTEMS

The practice of reimbursement for health care by prospective payment systems—diagnosis-related groups or health maintenance organizations—has developed without adequate consideration for the requirements of modern cancer management. New technologies, such as computerized tomography (CT) or magnetic resonance imaging (MRI) scanning, may be discouraged by the payment systems, although they improve care for patients. Payment is frequently denied for new anticancer drugs or treatments, even when the results are superior or cost effective.

The development of DRGs for Medicare inpatient payment was based on inadequate data to establish many of the cancer groups. For example, under the DRG system, acute leukemia in adults was allocated an inappropriately short length of inpatient care considering the seriousness of the illness and the intensity of supportive care required. Table 12.1 depicts the results of a survey by the Clinical Practice Committee of the American Society of Clinical Oncology (ASCO) of 16 selected cancer treatment facilities after the first year of prospective payment by DRGs. All leukemia and lymphoma DRGs were reviewed, accounting for 2,926 Medicare admissions from 9 university hospitals and 11 community hospitals.

The Health Care Financing Administration projected a 7.1 day median length of stay for Medicare DRG 403, the category used to describe acute leukemia or lymphomas treated with chemotherapy. The discrepancy between the actual length of stay for DRG 403 and the Medicare expected figure is significant: 11.6 days versus 7.1 days. Significant financial losses were incurred by every institution under DRG 403, as listed in Table 12.2. An average loss of $2,951 per admission under DRG 403 was reported

Table 12.1: Length of Stay for Leukemia-Lymphoma DRGs (in days)

DRG	Number of Admissions (University/Community)	Median Medicare LOS	Observed Average LOS	University Hospital LOS	Community Hospital LOS
400 Leukemia/lymphoma. major OR	154 (97/57)	16.9	12.3	15.2	11.9
401 Leukemia/lymphoma. minor OR, >69, or complication	136 (87/49)	8.9	10.8	13.3	10.0
402 Leukemia/lymphoma. minor OR, <70	35 (25/10)	7.1	5.0	4.5	10.0
403 Lymphoma/leukemia. >65 and/or complication	1,009 (773/276)	7.1	11.6	12.1	11.6
404 Lymphoma/leukemia. 18–69. without complication	135 (67/68)	6.4	5.0	4.0	7.0
405 Lymphoma/leukemia. 0–17	14	4.9	4.1	4.1	4.5
410 Chemotherapy	1,456 (740/716)	2.6	2.6	3.3	2.4

Source: Survey results of 2,926 Medicare admissions by the Clinical Practice Committee of the American Society for Clinical Oncology.

Notes: DRG = Diagnosis-Related Group; LOS = Average Length of Stay; OR = Operating Room Procedure.

Table 12.2: Average Losses or Gains by Leukemia-
Lymphoma DRG

DRG	Charge/ Patient	Loss or Gain per Patient	University Hospital	Community Hospital
400	$11,231	$ – 389	$ – 446	$ – 291
401	6,340	– 1,504	– 1,753	– 1,062
402	3,104	– 868	– 36	– 2,948
403	8,320	– 2,951	– 2,861	– 3,190
404	2,803	880	1,825	– 234
410	2,210	– 399	– 592	– 17

Note: Losses (– sign) or gains based on Medicare charges allowed and average
of surveyed costs by leukemia-lymphoma DRG as reported by university or
community hospitals. DRG 405 had an insufficient number of cases.

because of the underestimation of the care necessary for these ill
patients. Other DRG groupings represented average losses of $36
to $2,948, while DRG 404, uncomplicated lymphoma and leuke-
mias in adults, showed a net gain of $1,825 for university hospi-
tals in this sample.

The DRGs for lymphomas (400 – 405) represent a more heterogeneous group of diseases, which are classified by surgical procedures rather than by the severity of illness or care provided.
Diagnosis-related groups based on the actual care delivered or the
intensity of the illness would be more descriptive for the practice of
oncology. The ASCO has submitted data and proposals to change
the DRG descriptions to the Prospective Payment Assessment
Commission (PRoPAC) and HCFA, but only minor refinements
have been implemented. DRG 410, which was intended to
describe an admission for chemotherapy administration, is the
least expensive ($2,210 average charge) with the briefest hospital
stays (2.6 days expected). Medicare reviewers are assigning an
increasing number of patients within a heterogeneous group of
cancer diagnoses to DRG 410. Joanna Lion, of the Health Policy
Center of the Heller Graduate School of Brandeis University, has
published data showing that more cancer admissions are being
shifted to DRG 410 (Lion et al. 1987). The prospective payment
system, therefore, has been implemented so that it underfinances
complex medical care by placing cases in a simpler, less expensive
DRG group.

Cancer patients received more chemotherapy as outpatients
because admission criteria have become more rigid and technology has advanced to allow safe and comfortable administration

out of the hospital. Outpatients can receive chemotherapy at substantial cost savings, according to reports by Lion et al. (1987) and Prager (1984). Improved facilities for the preparation and administration of chemotherapy and better training for oncology nurses have made the quality of outpatient treatment equal or superior to inpatient care. Payment for these outpatient chemotherapy services under Medicare (Part B) is often inadequate, however, because state carriers do not cover the full cost of the drugs or the actual costs of administering the agents. Studies should be initiated to determine the actual costs of outpatient drug administration and to correct the underpayment of chemotherapy services. Chemotherapy agents must be fairly reimbursed by Medicare carriers.

Medical oncologists are discouraged from practicing in the most cost-effective or convenient way because of the inequities in the Medicare system. They are forced to admit patients for chemotherapy or to refer them to more expensive hospital-based outpatient units, because reimbursement is poor for these services when they are provided in physicians' offices. Members of ASCO report that they have stopped administering chemotherapy to Medicare patients in their offices because of the losses they incur. The ASCO would prefer to see incentives for physicians to provide efficient, humane care for cancer outpatients, and is working to communicate these goals to HCFA and to Congress.

RESEARCH AND NEW TECHNOLOGY

Perhaps no other area of medicine includes such widespread involvement in and commitment to clinical research as does oncology. Every university medical center has its clinical trials and cooperates with affiliates in outlying hospitals. Many oncologists participate in national cooperative treatment groups or community cancer outreach programs (CCOPs) designed to win the war against cancer.

Many clinical trials are limited because private and government health care providers have restricted payment for investigational patient care. The shortsighted approach of denying payment for care provided by a research program, just because it is ''investigational,'' is unfortunate. New and innovative approaches to cancer care, which may allow patients to be cured or remain active as wage earners, may be discouraged by such restrictions in payment. Prospective payment systems may dissuade oncologists from considering investigational programs for these patients if they know that payment may be denied or limited. The American Society of Clinical Oncology has suggested changes in health care payment by regulatory agencies that would encourage rather than discourage peer-reviewed clinical investigation.

Health maintenanace organizations that control costs by utilizing the gatekeeper mechanism of patient referral often limit access to the best medical specialty care. If financial considerations are part of the decision to refer to an oncologist or other specialist, patients may be denied necessary consultation. Close attention to quality and access to appropriate consultants in managed health care programs are essential. Medical specialty organizations have organized a coalition to work toward preserving the high quality of care we expect in the United States.

New techniques for the evaluation of cancer patients include CT scans, MRI scans, and monoclonal antibody diagnostic tests. Innovative chemotherapies and the highly publicized biologic response modifiers are under careful study so they can be rapidly introduced into the marketplace. Health care providers have no way to realistically evaluate or determine which techniques to pay for or to consider standard practice. The ASCO's Clinical Practice Committee is developing technology assessment mechanisms with the American Medical Association to provide assistance and expert advice to the health care industry.

THE FUTURE

Reimbursement for the care provided to cancer patients should be based on data that appropriately classify oncology practices and account for the intensity of care provided. Studies of modern treatments are critical in updating DRGs. If oncologists are expected to provide chemotherapy and other complicated services to outpatients, they must be fairly reimbursed. Poorly contrived plans such as DRGs are impossible to implement without a more comprehensive data base that reflects actual practice in the 1980s. The resource-based Relative Value Scale for physician payment, which is under study by the Harvard School of Public Health and the American Medical Association, may be more descriptive of the cognitive skills and the intensity of services provided. Specialty groups must be given an opportunity to participate in the development of such a new physician payment scale.

It is imperative that investigators evaluate the cost implications of new diagnostic techniques or treatment regimens, as well as the standard medical criteria. We need to assess the effect of our tests or therapies on the quality of life, as well as the length of survival or the shrinkage of tumor masses. Cancer researchers must consider the economic implications of their work so that new treatments can be appropriately represented to health care providers.

The health care industry should broaden its acceptance of clinical investigation by demanding the use of peer-reviewed clinical trials as the state of the art. Well-designed oncology research provides the highest quality of care, which is now often shunned because health insurers deny payment.

Physicians must insist on evaluating health care programs by the quality of the care provided and must develop standards by which to measure oncology care. We have the responsibility to assess new technologies prospectively, so that those that are productive can be rapidly accepted and covered by reimbursement mechanisms.

The physician perspective needs to be expanded beyond medical evaluation. We have to consider patient, hospital, insurer, and governmental perspectives in our established and new cancer management programs. A dialogue between all of these groups is essential to develop realistic cost control and still maintain high standards of cancer care. The ASCO and the American Cancer Society should work together with the health care industry to emphasize the importance of quality oncology care in a cost-conscious society.

REFERENCES

Lion, J.; Henderson, M.; Malbon, A.; and Berman, A. (1987). "Case Mix and Charges for Inpatient and Outpatient Chemotherapy." *Health Care Financing Review* 8(4): 65 – 71.

Prager, D. (1984). "Chemotherapy in the Physician's Office." *Pennsylvania Medicine* 37: 50 – 52.

13 Perspectives on the Issues: Cancer Centers

Richard J. Steckel

ABSTRACT.   Reimbursement for patient care, as a component of clinical cancer research, is an increasing problem at cancer centers throughout the country. With the exception of a few freestanding centers that have been exempted from the diagnosis-related group reimbursement mechanism by the Health Care Finance Administration, cancer research centers are now subject to fixed patient care payments which equate these institutions with nonresearch hospitals in the community. Since the "patient mix" in cancer research centers is skewed toward patients who are more difficult to treat, and since cost shifting to other sources for the in-hospital care of research patients is no longer allowable, most cancer research centers are finding it increasingly difficult to support their complex missions in clinical research, professional education, and state-of-the-art patient care.

This chapter considers the broad issues of reimbursement for patient care in connection with patient research, particularly as these issues pertain to cancer centers. Reimbursement issues in clinical research are becoming much more serious as time goes on, and they cry out for resolution before cancer research is severely curtailed.

Cancer research centers that receive core grant support from the National Cancer Institute are of several different types. Comprehensive cancer centers are broad-based programs in research, community outreach, education, and clinical care. Other types of centers include clinical cancer centers, which conduct predominantly clinical care and research, and basic cancer research centers, which do predominantly laboratory research. The prototype comprehensive cancer center, which existed before the National Cancer Act was passed in 1971, was Sloan Kettering-Memorial, which is a freestanding center. Most of the comprehensive and clinical cancer centers that have been organized with NCI core support since passage of the National Cancer Act, however, have been closely associated with universities and have *not* been freestanding (e.g., UCLA's Jonsson Comprehensive Cancer Center). In a few instances, quasi-independent units designated as cancer centers have been created within a university setting, with their own hospital and laboratory facilities (e.g., the Norris Cancer Research Institute at the University of Southern California, or the Dana Farber Center at Harvard).

The Health Care Financing Administration has granted a limited number of exemptions to the diagnosis-related group mechanism for freestanding cancer research centers, as well as for several quasi-independent cancer centers that have separate cancer hospitals and are located at university medical centers. However, other cancer centers that are supported by NCI, which have inpatient facilities that are closely integrated within their parent university hospitals, have not been provided with such exemptions. These constitute the majority of the NCI cancer centers that care for patients. While hard data are not yet available to indicate the impact of the two different reimbursement mechanisms (DRG versus fee-for-service) upon (1) patient care, and (2) patient-related research at the various types of cancer centers (Antman, Schnipper, and Frei 1988), there is obvious potential for creating a substantial economic advantage for those institutions that have a DRG exemption. Presumably, the latter institutions will continue to obtain a clinical reimbursement from government sources and third-party carriers on a fee-for-service basis.

Regardless of the mechanism used for clinical reimbursement, however, it is clear that both government and private third-party payers now intend to restrict patient care reimbursements to those costs that are strictly service related. Until now, there has been no doubt that some of the costs for patient care that were related to research protocols were shifted to government or private insurers, or to the patients themselves. Partial shifting of patient research costs to clinical care reimbursement sources is becoming increasingly difficult, however, and health care institutions themselves are also becoming more vigilant in preventing their patient care resources from being tapped to cover research costs. The apparent reluctance of government sponsors, such as Medicare and Medicaid, to provide full reimbursement for the services delivered by physicians-in-training at educational institutions has introduced additional difficulties for academic cancer centers, whose missions include not only research and patient care but professional education as well.

While there seems to be little choice left for cancer centers but to institute rigorous controls of their own in allocating costs between the different components of their mission (e.g., patient care, education, and research), there is still continuing disagreement between research institutions and the various patient care reimbursement sources (governmental as well as private) regarding the appropriate levels of payment for cancer care. Clearly, the patient mix at centers that carry out advanced cancer research and related teaching activities is not the same as the mix at many community care institutions, and DRG payments that are based upon the "average" patient with a specified medical condition cannot be assumed (necessarily) to be adequate for patients at tertiary care institutions, where the most difficult cases are often referred for treatment.

This is *not* tantamount to saying that a large proportion of the costs for research and professional training should be borne by third-party payers or by other patient care reimbursement sources. However, cancer patients with the most difficult clinical management problems in different DRG categories tend to be referred to cancer research centers, and therefore patient selection alone can be highly disadvantageous to centers when clinical care is reimbursed through non – fee-for-service mechanisms that are based upon "standard" costs of care in the community. Cancer centers that do research are not the only institutions struggling with this problem, since it is widely encountered by academic medical centers throughout the country. Except for the relatively few freestanding centers that initially received exemptions from the DRG mechanism, cancer centers that attract patients with conditions that are the most difficult to treat will be placed at an increasing disadvantage, unless durable solutions are found to their special problems of meeting patient care costs. Without such solutions, which recognize their unusual patient mix and their social contributions, cancer research centers will have great difficulty surviving, and prepayment and other fixed payment mechanisms will become the dominant methods of patient care reimbursement.

REFERENCE

Antman, D.; Schnipper, L. E.; and Frei, E. (1988) "Sounding Board—The Crisis in Clinical Cancer Research." *New England Journal of Medicine* 319(1): 46 – 48.

Part V

The Future of Financing Cancer Care

In 1987, health care expenditures in the United States exceeded $500 billion, a record high. Health care expenditures continue to rise at more than twice the rate of inflation (*San Francisco Chronicle*, 19 November 1988). The proposals that are adopted to control these costs in the future will have an important impact on health care, especially cancer care. Will cost-containment efforts be able to slow the rise in health care expenditures? What are the implications for the future of financing cancer care? These important questions are addressed from three different perspectives in Part V.

Chapters 14 and 15 are written from the perspective of nonprofit and private insurers. Leonard D. Schaeffer and Brian S. Gould, of Blue Cross of California, and David J. Ottensmeyer and M. K. Key, of EQUICOR, discuss the future role of the insurer in cancer care financing. Insurers face the dilemma of the need to constrain the high costs of cancer care without compromising the quality of care. To do this, insurers have shifted their focus from the financing mechanisms of health care to managing the delivery system itself. The managed care approach, including a broader system of ambulatory services, appears promising for serious chronic illnesses such as cancer. The authors conclude that, in order to be successful, cost containment will require partnerships between insurers, providers, payers, and individuals.

The third perspective examines cancer care from a societal perspective. Wilbur J. Cohen was one of the principle architects of the safety net system, consisting of Social Security, Medicare, and Medicaid. He was scheduled to speak at the 1987 American Cancer Society conference from which this book was conceived, but, unfortunately, he passed away before that time. His work is being carried out by Lonna T. Milburn, the contributor of Chapter 16. Cohen envisioned a universal, nationwide health care system, which would provide rights to both a full range of services and a high quality of health care, irrespective of race, age, gender, income, or national origin. Milburn examines this vision as it relates to cancer care. She points out that this dream has not been realized and that financial and organizational barriers to cancer care remain. She argues that a growing movement to restructure our nation's health care system could ultimately facilitate our nation's goal of reducing cancer incidence and mortality.

14 Cancer Care and Cost: The Blue Cross of California Approach

**Leonard D. Schaeffer and
Brian S. Gould**

ABSTRACT.   Cancer care represents the second largest expenditure category for Blue Cross of California. Although services are now being financed predominantly through HMO and PPO benefit plans, it is not yet evident that either type of organization has had a significant impact on cancer costs, or altered cancer's customary pattern of health care services. Case management programs, on the other hand, have been shown to influence expensive cases, but in cancer care they have been limited primarily to home hospice services as an alternative to hospital care in terminal cases. Additional development of "managed care" structural approaches, including a broader system of ambulatory cancer care services (particularly for maintenance chemotherapy), will be required before large-scale improvements in cancer treatment cost-effectiveness are realized. The expected benefits of managed care programs over conventional therapies are not limited to financial control, but extend to clinical and psychological improvements as well.

As the largest insurance carrier in the state, Blue Cross of California receives a large number of cancer-related claims reflecting a range in treatment from the most typical office visits to the most advanced methods and technology available in clinical medicine.

The important issue of how to finance the considerable costs of cancer care has three major areas of interest for consideration:

1. The financing mechanism currently being used to pay for cancer care
2. The types of care that are most expensive and why
3. Recommendations for changes in the financing mechanism that would improve the delivery of care to cancer patients without compromising quality

HOW IS CANCER CARE FINANCED CURRENTLY?

The best approach to this question is to examine cancer as a prototypical example of any major illness covered under Blue Cross insurance programs. As such, cancer care services are covered by benefits under one of three different basic mechanisms for health care financing: fee for service, preferred provider organizations, and health maintenance organizations.

Fee for Service

Sometimes referred to as "traditional insurance," this is the type that is probably most familiar to subscribers and providers. It is also sometimes referred to as "indemnity" insurance because it is built around a system of retrospective payment for covered billed services. Insurance carriers "indemnify" the subscriber against a portion of the financial obligation for medically necessary services (on a per service basis).

Because cancer is always a serious diagnosis, cancer care that is within the community standard of practice is virtually always a covered benefit of Blue Cross policies. Until recently, the only common area of controversy occurred when desperate members sought nonstandard and unapproved cancer treatments and wanted them covered by their insurance. With increasing experience with this clinical problem, Blue Cross contract language has become increasingly explicit regarding the limitation on therapies that fall outside the bounds of the community standard of medical practice. Generally, enforcement is a relatively straightforward matter (although this may be changing, as discussed below).

Preferred Provider Organizations

Approximately 50 percent of Blue Cross of California's members are now enrolled in PPO programs. This means that they receive a higher level of benefits for utilizing physicians and hospitals with whom Blue Cross has negotiated contracts, and for cooperating with utilization control programs such as preadmission certification, second surgical opinions, and case management. These two innovations, differential benefit levels and utilization controls, distinguish PPOs from indemnity coverage.

Here, too, the needs of cancer patients remain clinically consistent with the financing model. In the state's metropolitan areas we have been able to negotiate contracts with the major oncology resources and tertiary centers, so maintaining patients who require advanced medical services within the existing provider networks has not proved problematic. Although utilization review (UR) programs must monitor elective care against medical necessity standards, the clinical circumstances characteristic of cancer care lend themselves to this approach without exceptional difficulty. Because the diagnosis of most cancers is objectively verifiable, and treatment responses are usually already being monitored quantitatively by the clinical centers themselves, UR programs differentiate medically appropriate treatments from unnecessary or ineffective ones without frequent disputes.

Case management, which establishes an administrative-clinical team for complex, chronic, or otherwise expensive cases, is another major component of PPO cost control. Surprisingly, it appears to be of less benefit in cancer care than one would suppose. Its major application has been limited to terminal disease that is only "case managed" in the end stage of the illness (substituting hospice or home care for hospitalization). The underlying problem is the general lack of available alternative services during the lengthy course of cancer treatment. This is an example of how the PPO financing model does not necessarily result in substantial cost differences, because the pattern of services for many patients remains unchanged.[1]

Health Maintenance Organizations

During the 1980s, California experienced an astounding level of enrollment migration from traditional insurance programs to health maintenance organizations. In some parts of the state, fully 40 percent of the insured population are now members of these capitated, highly directed programs.[2]

Because HMO provider networks are more restricted than those of PPOs, and because their out-of-network benefits are far more limited, it is possible that a distinguishably different pattern of services for treating cancer in capitated environments will develop. So far, however, hard data have not supported that prediction.[3] Rates and timing of diagnosis; selection and duration of treatments; and mortality and morbidity rates do not seem to be significantly variant under different insurance models (when the population at risk is age adjusted).

It should be noted that approximately 10 percent of Blue Cross total claims costs (company-wide, all programs) are for cancer care, without significant differences attributable to the insurance financing model.

WHICH TYPES OF CARE ARE THE MOST EXPENSIVE AND WHY?

Generally speaking, the expense of medical treatment correlates directly with the level of resource consumption. Typically, this means diseases that cause high utilization of hospital services or require high-technology treatment interventions cost more to treat regardless of site. Not surprisingly, Blue Cross considers cancer an "expensive" illness.[4] High-technology diagnostic imaging, isotope scanning, multiple surgeries, radiotherapy, recurrent hospitalizations, transfusions, and expensive courses of chemotherapy are all common services in the longitudinal course of cancer care.

Further, cancer is relatively unusual in that it often requires treatment that causes a high level of iatrogenic morbidity (which then must also be treated). This factor alone would push cancer into the ranks of high-cost illnesses, even if cancer primary care was not particularly resource consumptive.

An additional development that threatens to push up the average cost of cancer care even further is the gradual obscuring of the all-important coverage boundary between investigational treatments and accepted medical practices.

The pace of medical technological transfer is continually accelerating, with almost immediate communication of recent advances to the physician community and even to the general public. It is not uncommon for the *New England Journal of Medicine* to carry a brief research report that is picked up by local newspapers and immediately described as a treatment option to insured patients. (On more than one occasion, Blue Cross has been requested to pay for patients who were participating in a research study and might have been receiving placebo treatment!)

While the ethics of clinical practice may encourage the use of all possible treatment alternatives in otherwise hopeless situations, the practical impact of this response, from a health economics perspective, is usually to increase the cost of an inevitably fatal outcome. In other words, pursuing ineffective treatments in hopeless situations has the effect of increasing the eventual cost of dying—now estimated to be as much as $80,000 in the United States.[5]

For example, there is a trend toward recommending autologous bone marrow transplantation (ABMT) for relapsing cancers of assorted types. This dangerous and expensive technique has demonstrated effectiveness for specific cancers, particularly lymphomas and leukemias, but remains totally investigational in all other circumstances. Yet despite ABMT's considerable risks and expense, and despite a conspicuous absence of efficacy data, Blue Cross has received a cascade of claims for ABMT in other cancers. For the patient losing her battle with breast cancer, ABMT's known resistance to this approach is no reason not to want to try it. But was this the purpose of the insurance? Did the premiums anticipate this expense? Does this mean that the insurer must fund any treatment attempt, no matter how expensive or unscientific, if the situation is desperate enough?

The traditional exclusion of coverage for experimental treatments is being challenged, therefore, not on the basis of safety and effectiveness, which one would prefer, but instead on the emotional level of the situation and the state of public opinion regarding the technique. Can we continue to classify a treatment as investigational if it lacks supporting scientific evidence, but is nonetheless utilized frequently? American medicine soundly rejected this argument when it was used to support Laetrile, but seems much more tolerant to clinical faddishness when it involves higher technology.

In the meantime, the financial implication of an unscientific "last ditch" treatment attempt that adds $100,000 to each breast cancer death is staggering. And as the public becomes aware of these treatment fads, it becomes more and more difficult for even responsible physicians to refuse the ineffective treatment to any patient who demands it. In time, the basic financial integrity of the medical care plan is jeopardized.

WHAT CHANGES IN FINANCING MECHANISMS WOULD IMPROVE THE DELIVERY OF SERVICE TO CANCER PATIENTS WITHOUT REDUCING QUALITY?

Blue Cross approaches the future with the following basic premises:

1. Cancer is an increasingly *treatable* disease.
2. The costs associated with its treatment are already considerable, and likely to continue to increase with progress in medical technology.
3. These costs cannot be entirely eliminated, but can be controlled by adopting treatment strategies that make cost-effectiveness a priority for the delivery system.

Therefore, the Blue Cross of California policy development strategy has shifted its focus from the financial mechanisms of health care to managing the delivery system itself. The most appropriate challenge for the future is to improve outcomes for people with legitimate medical needs, at the same time as costs are being controlled (i.e., to strive to improve cost-effectiveness rather than simply reduce costs).

The successful delivery system for cancer care will need to

- eliminate unnecessary care,
- reduce encounters,
- reduce the need for hospital admissions and length of stay associated with routine treatments,
- reduce the level of iatrogenic morbidity associated with cancer treatment,
- reduce administrative costs,
- assist psychosocial adjustment to cancer and cancer treatment, and
- improve clinical outcomes.

Historically, Blue Cross has had generally poor results with cost-containment programs because the approach has been exclusively financial, focusing either on the costs per unit of care, the number of units consumed, or on benefit incentives to direct the patient's choice of provider. This approach no longer seems adequate to gain control of the cost problem over the long run, or to achieve the clinical objectives listed above.

Carriers are moving away from a posture of passively and retrospectively paying for whatever medical services have been delivered (even at a discount); they are moving toward a system in which all players agree to manage a course of treatment in the least expensive way for the benefit of the patient. The current descriptive term for this approach is "managed care." In this context, "management" implies the existence of an *organized system* that can act to achieve an optimum level of efficiency and productivity, and possesses the capability to influence the physical reality of *how* services are delivered to achieve these results.

Blue Cross views the future for large carriers as clearly shifting from traditional insurance functions to these managed care programs, and the company expects to explore the application of industrial management science to health care delivery. The current levels of waste and inefficiency in health care make this a tempting target. Although it has not provided all of the answers, the application of management science to health care delivery has raised some interesting questions.

For example, in the complex modern health care system, what levels of management control are necessary, and who is best situated to fulfill the managerial role for optimum results? To put the same question in somewhat different terminology, can we redefine the roles and interrelationships of the carrier, the providers, the payers (and their brokers and consultants), and the beneficiaries (and their families) to promote more cost-effective system operations and behaviors?

The initial conceptualization of such a system emphasizes the complementary responsibilities of these agents functioning in the roles of (1) system manager (carrier); (2) care managers (providers, primarily physicians); (3) resource manager (payer); and (4) individual managers (referring to the beneficiary/patient's responsibility in maintaining his or her own health, choosing between alternative treatments, and adhering to the demands of the treatment plan selected).

Cancer care tends to be distinctly *unlike* the hypothetical, unspecified illness used in health planning, according to the principles of cost containment. In such scenarios we can, for example, reliably produce considerable cost savings by shifting a single surgical procedure from an inpatient to an outpatient setting. But cancer care rarely involves a single, simple surgery capable of being handled on a "come and go" basis. Rather, it is much more

common for a course of cancer treatment to require ongoing combinations of major techniques, such as surgery, radiation, and
chemotherapy.

In addition, cancer care is atypical in that outcomes are not a
generally reliable basis for monitoring treatment. "Good treatment" cannot be judged solely on the basis of whether or not the
patient is responding. Good treatments can be associated with
poor outcomes, and remissions are not necessarily the result of
early treatment. Even when remissions are successfully achieved
as the result of treatment, they may not be permanent, nor are
they a justification for the cessation of treatment. On the other
hand, relapses can be regular, even expected, events that do not
necessarily reflect inadequate treatment or poor prognosis. Even
the most successfully treated cancer patient may go on to suffer
occurrences of additional tumors of a different type after the primary disease is in remission.

In short, at the current level of medical science, "cancer"
generally means a chronic recurrent illness requiring an extended
course of treatment, regardless of the initial response. Therefore,
the application of managed care to cancer care will require simul-
taneous concern with the inescapable disease characteristics of
high average service unit costs combined with high aggregate episode costs. However, it is exactly this type of illness pattern in
which early managed care approaches have had their greatest
impact. It is only in serious chronic illnesses that careful management of health care services can demonstrate its advantages.[6]

A "successful outcome" in cancer treatment, as most people
would define it, is never a matter of a simple statistical survival
rate. Quality of life is of far greater importance than length of survival to most individuals. This perception includes more subtle
dimensions, such as level of comfort and relief of pain; personal
level of control over the environment; level of preserved or restored
function; and most importantly, the ability to maintain and
remain active in significant interpersonal relationships.

We should recognize that in the eyes of most people, the most
successful cancer care outcomes would actually be *more* achievable in noninstitutional settings. Home care and other so-called
alternative treatments are not only potentially more cost effective,
as measured by direct biological outcome parameters, but are also
associated with this greater sense of treatment success for most
individuals who appreciate their ability to remain functional and
active at home and among their own people.

An example of this type of approach is the pilot program now being conducted by a hospital in Los Angeles for the extended treatment of leukemia on an outpatient basis. Patients in this program can often undergo complete courses of chemotherapy without requiring *any* inpatient confinement, except in cases of severe morbidity. This is achieved through a carefully planned and coordinated multimodality treatment strategy; a much higher level of patient and family education, allowing them to assume a more sophisticated role in self-care; and the application of a key new technology: the ambulatory portable intravenous pump. In this way, technology that ironically has a significantly greater unit cost is applied in the delivery system, so that its potential for much greater overall treatment cost-effectiveness is achieved.

Such care is still relatively expensive, and out-of-area patients will still need to reside in local hotels, but there is no question that the comparative episode costs and total costs are significantly lower than standard care for the same conditions.[7] Perhaps more importantly, the patient and family never experience the feelings of surrender of personal control to the illness and to the health care providers that have historically been among the most feared consequences of cancer. This has been described by those who have experienced it as one of the most damaging losses caused by the disease.

Instead of surrendering into passivity, patients in this environment are actively mobilized by the educational process that incorporates them and their families into a treatment team that includes the physicians, nurses, family therapists, social workers, and health educators. The higher level of patient involvement and activism also carries over to their home when the patients leave the clinic-centered treatment. At this point, the patient's local physician (who has also been briefed on the patient's current status and prepared for the transfer home by the clinic staff) resumes a role on the extended treatment "team."

This approach to routine cancer care has generated growing enthusiasm. The program is expected to be successful because most patients are far more comfortable at home, and they do much better psychologically when the disruption to their ordinary life and relationships is minimized.[8] Therefore, assuming cancer care at home can be delivered in a manner that is equally medically efficacious, it would then be generally superior to hospital care in virtually all other respects.

In addition to the obvious advances in medical technology and delivery system coordination, note how many of the services associated with full ambulatory care would not have been covered adequately under traditional insurance benefits. In order for managed care to work, there must be coordinated development of the clinical, administrative, and financial formats. Among Blue Cross's responsibilities in improving health care is the job of making sure innovative managed care approaches are covered appropriately in future programs.

Blue Cross sees the keys to this better future as the following:

- Insurance carriers should become more flexible and more involved in the direction of the extended delivery system.

- Providers should be more willing to plan and manage treatment programs so that individual outcomes are optimized for cost-effectiveness, and limited resources are marshalled for greatest impact.

- Payers should become more willing to fund nontraditional benefit designs that promote greater levels of cost-effectiveness of overall care.

- Individuals should prepare themselves for, and then take on a greater level of responsibility for, their own health care.

NOTES

1. The considerable publicity that has trumpeted the putative cost-containment features of PPOs (such as discounted hospital and professional fees, and restrictions on elective hospital utilization) has tended to obscure the realization that despite the innovation of contract-based service delivery, this model continues to *preserve* fee-for-service incentives in selecting treatment approaches, and that we know less about its performance under real life conditions than we should.

   Diehr (1987) demonstrates that the ambulatory costs for a Uniformed Services population were lower in a PPO environment than under a pure fee-for-service insurance program, but were not as low as a comparison closed-panel HMO. Unfortunately, this finding could not be connected to any measurement of overall cost-effectiveness (are lower ambulatory costs better or worse in terms of total plan cost?), nor could the authors control for the factor that this population habitually used more health services in absolute terms than the general population.

   A most significant observation was made by Wouters and Hester (1988), whose study appears to demonstrate a somewhat reduced level of utilization in the PPO. However, the authors caution that, rather than reflecting more cost-effective service delivery, there are indications that the PPO system was preferentially "selected by individuals who require relatively little medical care."

One must conclude that the impact of this financial design on health service patterns is still an open question.

2. The annual survey of HMO activity compiled by SMG Marketing Group, Chicago, indicates that in 1987, 61 HMOs were state-qualified for operation in California (the largest number nationally, and a 34 percent increase from 1986), with a 27.7 percent penetration of the state's population (16.2 percent increase in enrollment compared to 1986). Since only a portion of the state population is covered by private insurance, this represents an incredible growth in the real market penetration of HMO programs.

3. Francis, Polissar, and Lorenz (1984) observed a somewhat delayed interval between first physician encounter and treatment in the HMO group. However, there were no significant differences in other dimensions of care such as accessibility, treatment type, length of hospital stay, or four-year survival rates. McCusker, Stoddard, and Sorensen (1988) repeated this finding in a matched-pair comparison of terminal patients (deaths occurring 1976 – 82.) Although their HMO group used fewer hospital days and had somewhat lower costs, neither difference reached statistical significance.

4. Justifying the use of relative terms such as "expensive" through a quantitative process is, alas, always open to dispute. Nevertheless, cancer-identified claims have been shown to represent a significant proportion of Blue Cross of California's annual aggregate claims expense. For the under-65 individual and small group market, this segment represents between 9 and 10 percent of the Blue Cross total claims cost—the second highest grouping, exceeded only by all accidents and injuries (14 percent), and about equal to all maternity and newborn expenses.

Lansky (1987) presents a more subjective treatment of this subject.

5. This is a figure one frequently hears quoted at industry gatherings such as business round tables. As is so often the case with conventional wisdom, it is difficult to find unequivocal support for the actual number in the scientific literature.

Riley et al. (1987) indicate that enrollees in the last year of life account for "over one-fourth of total medical expenditures." Cancer was the most expensive leading cause of death, but per capita expenses are cited as averaging only $8,021. This is curious because the McCusker study focused on the same approximate time frame and indicated that the non-HMO cancer deaths averaged more than $9,000 each for hospital costs alone and only for the last six months of life, rather than twelve (McCusker, Stoddard, and Sorensen 1988). (This was at a time and for a group in which the average hospital day rate was only $325. At today's average rates the same utilization pattern would be about $28,000 for hospital charges alone.)

Cohn (1984) quotes a 1981 study at Peter Bent Brigham Hospital that randomly identified 36 high-cost cases that were determined in follow-up to have been terminal. Prior to dying, however, these relatively few individuals required nearly $2,000,000 of care (or $55,555 each).

6. Again, it is difficult to estimate quantitatively the extent of the payoff. In experience with case management in several other illnesses (specifically AIDS, head and spinal cord injuries, and neonatal complications), Blue Cross of California has realized an average savings range of $15,000 – $35,000 per case when we have been allowed to assist the organization of treatment resources. Restricting treatment services per se is not a goal of case management.

For several reasons, case management in cancer care has been essentially limited to terminal rather than ongoing care, and instances where hospice and home care can be substituted for the final hospital confinement. While this approach is undeniably cost effective (Gray, MacAdam, and Boldy 1987), terminal care barely begins to exploit the potential for managed care techniques to achieve more rational allocation of treatment resources. Such demonstration will require the proliferation of more alternative treatment resources applied far earlier in the course of illness (Clark 1986).

7. Although one must be careful about extrapolating across national borders when it comes to health care financing, a Canadian study by Wodinsky et al. (1987) determined that chemotherapy administered at the Toronto-Bayview Regional Cancer Centre was 22 percent less expensive on a dose-for-dose basis (over six months) than identical protocols conducted at the Sunnybrook Medical Centre, Toronto. Since the actual "total cost" of inpatient administration was calculated to be only $185.39 per dose in this Canadian hospital, and the difference compared to outpatient treatment was "predominantly due to a higher allocated per-diem charge at the medical centre," we could expect a much more dramatic comparison in the United States system.

8. There is abundant and constantly updated literature on the subject of psychosocial adaptation to cancer. Resource articles range from comprehensive overview articles (Fawzy et al. 1983) to more focused treatments of the complex dynamics of social support during the phases of neoplastic illness (Wortman 1984).

In addition, although it was published in 1972, Avery Weisman's superb book, *On Dying and Denying*, is still worth rereading (Weisman 1972). It cautions that the disruption of personal relationships caused by severe illness causes more psychological distress "than does the specter of death itself." It is reasonable to predict that newer treatment strategies that minimize disruptions of identity and interpersonal and environmental supports would, in addition to providing direct physiologic benefits, assist in the psychological adjustment to illness with cancer.

REFERENCES

Clark, M. (1986). "A Day Hospital for Cancer Patients: Clinical and Economic Feasibility." *Oncological Nursing Forum* 13(November-December): 41 – 45.

Cohn, R. B. (1984). "The Inverse Relationship Between Cost and Prognosis." *Laryngoscope* 94(March): 340 – 42.

Diehr, P. (1987). "Use of Ambulatory Health Care Services in a Preferred Provider Organization." *Medical Care* 25(November): 1033 – 43.

Fawzy, F. I., et al. (1983). "Psychosocial Management of Cancer." *Psychiatric Medicine* 1(June): 165 – 80.

Francis, A. M.; Polissar, L.; and Lorenz, A. B. (1984). "Care of Patients with Colorectal Cancer: A Comparison of a Health Maintenance Organization and Fee-for-Service Practices." *Medical Care* 22(5): 418 – 29.

Gray, D.; MacAdam, D.; and Boldy, D. (1987). "A Comparative Cost Analysis of Terminal Cancer Care in Home Hospice Patients and Controls." *Journal of Chronic Diseases* 40(8): 801 – 10.

Lansky, S. B. (1987). "The High Cost of Cancer." *American Journal of Pediatric Hematology/Oncology* 9(Spring): 89 – 91.

McCusker, J.; Stoddard, A. M.; and Sorensen, A. A. (1988). "Do HMOs Reduce Hospitalization of Terminal Cancer Patients?" *Inquiry* 25(Summer): 263 – 70.

Riley, G.; Lubitz, J.; Prihoda, R.; and Rabey, E. (1987). "The Use and Costs of Medicare Services by Cost of Death." *Inquiry* 24(3): 233 – 44.

Weisman, A. (1972). *On Dying and Denying.* New York: Behavioral Publications.

Wodinsky, H. B.; De Angelis, C.; Rusthoven, J. J.; Kerr, I. G.; Sutherland, D.; Iscoe, N.; Buckman, R.; and Kornijenko, M. (1987). "Re-evaluating the Cost of Outpatient Cancer Chemotherapy." *Canadian Medical Association Journal* 137(November 15): 903 – 6.

Wortman, C. B. (1984). "Social Support and the Cancer Patient: Conceptual and Methodologic Issues." *Cancer* 53(10 Suppl.): 2339 – 62.

Wouters, A. V., and Hester, J. (1988). "Patient Choice of Providers in a Preferred Provider Organization." *Medical Care* 26(3): 240 – 55.

15 The Future of Financing Cancer Care: The Private Insurer's Viewpoint

David J. Ottensmeyer and M. K. Key

ABSTRACT.   Cancer is a catastrophic illness that affects the insured as well as the uninsured and the medically indigent. Private insurance is not designed to solve the social problem of making care available to a denied segment of our population. Among the mechanisms of indemnity, managed care, and employer self-funding, the real opportunity for savings exists in managed care—that is, the use of strategies such as medical management, "centers of excellence," and medical case management. The insurance mechanism cannot create new resources for cancer care, but through managed care, it can free up dollars that society may choose to spend on other problems of equity or access to cancer care.

THE PROBLEM

We are not doing very well in the war on cancer. Despite improvements in treatment, palliation, and extension of productive years of life, cancer is still on the rise. Age-adjusted mortality rates have shown a slow and steady increase over several decades, and there is no evidence of a downward trend (Bailer and Smith 1986). In fact, it appears that the incidence of cancer will continue to increase over the next 40 to 50 years; by the year 2030, the number of new cases per year may double, fueled by the population growth of the baby boom (Janerich 1984). Moreover, the per capita costs of cancer are increasing due not only to population growth, but also as a consequence of more expensive technologies and longer survival periods. Hospitals' future cancer inpatient load is estimated at 30 to 40 percent of the total general hospital patient population (measured by patient days) (Kenney 1986). Clearly, we must prepare for cancer's increasing presence among us and for the financing of cancer care.

Concern about health care expenditures swelled again in the mid-1980s, fueled by the AIDS crisis, the plight of the uninsured and underinsured, trends in the workplace (whereby one-half of the major employers have become self-insured), and the growing reluctance of employers and government to cover all costs of health care. While much of this discussion focuses on those without health insurance protection or the medically indigent, persons covered by private insurance are also affected. Seventy-three percent of individuals in the United States have private health insurance protection covering hospitalization, 80 percent if those 65 and over are included (based on 1984 statistics). The privately insured group is also subject to large out-of-pocket expenditures because of cost-sharing features, upper limits on their policies, or exclusions in coverage. The cost of intensive cancer care—particularly for the terminally ill—is a serious matter for patient and insurer alike.

THE ROLE OF PRIVATE INSURANCE

What is the role of insurance in dealing with catastrophic and deadly diseases? This is difficult to explain without first examining the insurance mechanism, which is based on the law of large numbers.

Insurance is designed to cover the possibility of loss due to a sudden and unexpected hazard beyond the control of the individual. It operates by spreading risk over large groups of people and actuarially determining the likelihood of catastrophic occurrences. The underlying premise is that only a few individuals will have catastrophic claims, as assessed from past experience. In essence, insurance seeks to predict the future by extrapolating from trends of the past. Under strict insurance principles, in order for the insurance mechanism to operate properly, (1) the extent of the loss must be measurable (of known cost proportions), and (2) the possibility of the loss to the individual must be uncertain (Lifson and Lieberman 1986).

Premiums are then determined by degree of risk, group characteristics, and market forces (e.g., what the competition is charging). At renewal, groups are rerated based on their previous experience, unless they have purchased pooling coverage (in the case of the fully insured) or stop-loss coverage (for the self-funded). Then claims above a predetermined point (e.g., $50,000) are generally not charged to a particular group but averaged over all insureds. In this manner, increases in dollar amounts of claims drive up premiums and the cost of insurance. Insurance cannot work without the ability to charge back costs in this manner.

Private insurance is *not designed* (although it has been used) to solve social problems, such as making care available to some denied segment of our population. It does not presume to improve the standard of living, nor is it calculated to solve massive health problems, such as the AIDS crisis. It is difficult to predict AIDS because we have insufficient experience; it is an undefined threat of the future. Without experience or trends, an insurance company has no way to set rates.

DIFFERENT INSURANCE PLANS

The known forms of cancer are predictable entities. For patients under 65, Blue Cross and private insurers are the source of payment for care in over 77 percent of the cases (American Cancer Society 1987). Funding for cancer treatment is derived from premium dollars paid, either on a capitation (per capita) or an indemnity (per service) basis. Under the traditional insurance plan, a subscriber typically meets a deductible amount, then makes copayments up to a maximum out-of-pocket amount, usually in the range of $1,000 to $3,000. A cap exists on total maximum coverage of an amount such as $1 million for a lifetime. In this way, the subscriber shares risk with the insurer and knows what their maximum out-of-pocket costs of major illness would be.

Alternately, managed health care plans may utilize capitation (prepayment of a flat fee per member per month) or discounted fee-for-service payment to the provider of service. The subscriber's cost does not change with the amount of services received and remains constant for a fixed period, usually one year. Deductibles and copayments are usually required. Under managed care, the plan is responsible for all medically necessary services to its enrollees. The insurance carrier arranges and manages a network of providers to deliver the health care services. The providers enter into risk/incentive arrangements with the insured, designed to reward quality and cost-effective care. The trend is away from traditional fee-for-service options, because the incentives are to generate more service, which generates more revenue for the provider and causes greater cost for the purchaser of the care (government, employers, and unions).

Prompted by potential cost savings and the 1974 passage of the Employee Retirement Income Security Act (ERISA), employers have increasingly elected to "self-fund" medical benefits for their employees and use the insurance company as the administrator of their benefits program. The insurance company simply writes checks on the employer's account. This "stop-loss" insurance is coverage that allows small- to medium-sized employers to self-fund part of their health benefits while transferring the risk of large medical claims to an insurer. The employer chooses a level at which specific stop-loss insurance takes over the cost of a case. Employers covering more than 2,000 lives usually do not purchase this kind of insurance, and the market for stop-loss is limited (Strazewski 1984). As stop-loss or excess insurance becomes less available, and employers suffer more catastrophic occurrences or risk (e.g., AIDS), they will confront the same issues of funding that insurance companies face.

CONTROLLING COSTS: MANAGED HEALTH CARE

The major issue facing any insurance plan is cost. Health care costs for the terminally ill cancer patient during the last six months of life average nearly $16,000 (Charles D. Spencer and Associates 1983). Insurance studies have shown that cancer care can average $53,109 per case, with cancer cases making up 11 percent of total nonmanaged claims (Equitable Life Assurance 1986). Hospital expenditures can account for 78 percent of the total cost of cancer care, with physicians' expenditures making up 16 percent (Charles D. Spencer and Associates 1983).

There is little evidence that we have done much to control costs. The only real opportunity left for continued cost savings is in the effective management of the delivery of health services. Managed health care can enhance our ability to control costs, by selecting providers and by controlling the quality, efficiency, and effectiveness of the systems that deliver care. Managed health care uses a variety of tools to control quality and efficiency of care. Two of the tools utilized in managed care are the "centers of excellence" concept and medical case management.

"Centers of excellence" is a concept utilized by government and private industry to concentrate business in the very best institutions for the purpose of excellence (e.g., with organ transplants). By focusing the maximum amount of expertise on high-cost health care problems, the cost balance can be favorably shifted so that there are more resources to go around. This prevents unnecessary duplication of equipment and services, low ratio of patients to providers and, therefore, low levels of practice experience that are not a concomitant of excellence.

Most of the major insurance carriers now offer medical case management (MCM) services. Even a major medical policy provides only partial protection against the costs of catastrophic illness. Months of intensive chemotherapy on a critical care unit may leave a patient exposed to unpredictably large financial burdens, after meeting deductible, coinsurance, and maximum reimbursement amounts. Traditional indemnity insurance covers only room and board plus ancillaries (e.g., tests, drugs). Although total cost savings may be realized when expensive inpatient cancer treatment is moved to an outpatient basis, there are often disincentives for the patient (Ward 1983). Out-of-pocket medical expenses, plus out-of-pocket nonmedical items (e.g., transportation, lodging), are not covered under typical indemnity plans. The very nature of that financing may force people to get a level of care not needed. Medical case management was created to manage that problem.

In the case of catastrophic illness, MCM can go outside of certain contractual provisions to provide for care that is medically necessary and appropriate, to manage limited dollars within the lifetime limit of the contract. The MCM approach is to mitigate medical costs by intervening early in the course of treatment and promoting the use of accelerated care (e.g., specialized rehabilitation), alternate care (e.g., home health care), and palliative care (e.g., home modifications). The MCM specialist in a given disease entity works on an individual basis with the patient, the patient's family, and the physician to intervene early enough for the most *care*-effective treatment—that is, care that optimizes the level of recovery and independence for those in rehabilitation or provides the optimal level of comfort and dignity for those who are terminally ill. In general, the care-effective options will also be the most cost effective.

Alternate modes of care in a less restrictive environment,

such as home or outpatient care, may lead to faster recovery for the patient and lower long-term costs. Accelerated care (specialized rehabilitation, more intensive therapies) and palliative care to prevent complications may realize further cost savings. Medical case management specialists coordinate services and resources (including facilities, equipment, training, family counseling, transportation, and professional and nonprofessional support networks), all of which are completely reimbursed. There is considerable evidence that case management can effectively lower costs for the patient, the employer, and the insurer (Clarke 1986; Eshelman 1986; Garner 1987; Lenkus 1986; Tonsfeldt 1986).

The two concepts—"centers of excellence" and MCM—bring the maximum amount of expertise to bear on unusual and high-cost problems. Health insurance companies use them to maximize the effectiveness of each available dollar provided by the contract.

THE FUTURE

Again, the question is: "What is the role of insurance in financing cancer care?" What is *really* the problem? It is the allocation of resources within society. There is not enough money to meet the needs of research, new technology, treatment, and the increasing incidence of cancer. If the ultimate cure for cancer is discovered tomorrow and it costs $1 million per individual, will policymakers or employers or private citizens pay? Who is the "they" that ought to pay? This is not simply an insurance problem, but a societal problem. The consumer of health care ultimately pays—in the form of premiums, taxes, or dollars devoted to health insurance premiums—dollars that would otherwise be available for other goods for society or the world.

There are no new resources created by insurance; inadequate resources for cancer treatment will compete and suffer trade-offs with therapy for AIDS, interventions to protect the elderly, or demand for expansion of national defense. If dollars are saved through managed health care, these dollars could go to cancer therapy. But if the dollars are diverted to other societal problems, or if business organizations retain the savings to enhance their bottom line, then there are no new dollars to finance cancer care. What insurance has to offer is the rating of experience, spreading of risk, and tight management of the care. The funding choices remain with society.

REFERENCES

American Cancer Society. (1987). *Cancer Facts and Figures—1987*. New York: American Cancer Society.

Bailer, J. C., and Smith, E. M. (1986). "Progress Against Cancer?" *New England Journal of Medicine* 314(19): 1226–32.

Charles D. Spencer and Associates. (1983). Study Investigates Costs of Various Cancer Treatments." *Employee Benefit Plan Review* 37(11): 100, 102.

Clarke, A. G. (1986). "10th Annual Eastern Claims Conference—AIDS—Only the Tip of the Iceberg?" *Best's Review* (Life/Health) 86(12): 131–32.

Equitable Life Assurance. (1986). "1984 Unmanaged Cancer Case Costs." Equitable Claims Study. Raw data.

Eshelman, C. (1986). "A Quick Fix Is No Cure for Rising Medical Benefit Costs." *Risk Management* 33(4): 54–60.

Garner, J. (1987). "Tailored Savings—Case Management Can Trim Companies' Health Care Costs." *Business Insurance* 21(6): 23–24.

Janerich, D. T. (1984). "Forecasting Cancer Trends to Optimize Control Strategies." *Journal of the National Cancer Institute* 72(6): 1317–21.

Kenney, A. (1986). "Outpatient Cancer Treatment Stresses Education." *American Medical News* 29(23): 19–20.

Lenkus, D. (1986). "Case Managers Can Cut Cost of Catastrophic Care: Experts." *Business Insurance* 20(7): 10–11.

Lifson, A., and Lieberman, P. (1986). "Insurance Coverage and AIDS." New York: Equitable Life Assurance.

Strazewski, L. (1984). "Stop-Loss Insurers Stung by High Health Costs." *Business Insurance* 18(5): 18, 20.

Tonsfeldt, L. (1986). "Cost Management through Case Management." *Personnel Journal* 65(3): 74–79.

Ward, W. J. (1983). "A Proposal for the Deinstitutionalization of Patients." *Health Care Management Review* 8(2): 73–77.

16 Cancer Care and Cost Beyond DRGs: A National Plan

Lonna T. Milburn

ABSTRACT. Overall, our present health care system receives relatively low marks for its impact on cancer care and costs. Financial and organizational barriers restrain individuals from seeking necessary cancer care. A growing movement to restructure our nation's health care system could ultimately facilitate our nation's goal to reduce cancer incidence and mortality. With a nationwide health plan, all U.S. citizens will be entitled to receive cancer care that best ensures their happiness and productivity.

Beyond diagnosis-related groups there must be a delivery and financing plan that thwarts cancer's deadly impact. While implementation of the DRG reimbursement method has initially influenced health care delivery and cut growing health care costs, it has only compromised the availability and quality of cancer care over the long term. Today, cancer care is jeopardized when breakdowns in DRG coverage discourage individuals from attending cancer prevention classes, visiting cancer diagnostic centers, or receiving proper cancer therapy. Once within the health care system, a patient might be discharged prematurely, denied access to necessary supplies, or left to initiate and monitor care singlehandedly. Therefore, our effectiveness in combating the cancer killer is threatened.

A review of cancer rate patterns shows that, in spite of improved preventive, diagnostic, and treatment methods, cancer

Table 16.1: Rate of Cancer per 100,000 Population, 1983–87

Year	All Ages	65–74 Years	75–84 Years	85+ Years
1983	188.3	831.7	1,227.6	1,610.5
1984	191.6	830.0	1,272.7	1,559.1
1985	193.3	837.8	1,261.9	1,569.4
1986	193.3	841.0	1,261.4	1,602.3
1987	196.1	845.8	1,282.8	1,631.7

continues to stalk the land with increasing intensity. Cancer deaths increased per 100,000 population from 188.3 in 1983 to 196.1 in 1987 (National Center for Health Statistics 1987a, 1987b, 1988). Cancer mortality rates for the population over 65 years show similar increases (Table 16.1). In 1988, some 985,000 Americans will be diagnosed with cancer and 494,000 will die of the disease (American Cancer Society 1988). Undoubtedly, this growing rate of cancer will continue unabated until our nation's health care system organizes its resources to deliver health care more efficiently and effectively.

A NATIONAL HEALTH PLAN

Beyond DRGs lies a system that has its roots in the social movement at the beginning of this century. In 1913, President Woodrow Wilson suggested that the U.S. health care system be organized and financed under a nationalized plan. The Wilson plan, along with countless other initiatives in the Franklin Roosevelt, Truman, Eisenhower, Nixon, and Carter administrations, lacked the necessary momentum for enactment. Typically, the fault was with powerful interest groups who claimed that a nationalized approach represented socialism, rigid regulation, and inflexible centralism (Morris 1984).

Today, a growing interest in a national health plan heralds the formation of health care coalitions dedicated to providing an all-American, universal health care service. Hundreds of diverse groups, representing health care, labor, education, and consumer advocates, are scrambling to define realistic parameters for such a system (Committee for a National Program 1987; Gray Panthers 1988; Frieda Wolff National Health Service Fund 1988; National Health Care Campaign 1987). In addition, several state governments are examining this universal concept for inclusion in a legislative package (Dallek, Hurwit, and Golde 1987). In 1988, after several unsuccessful attempts, Massachusetts became the first state to pass a statewide universal plan (Massachusetts Commonwealth 1988).

Several points are basic to the Massachusetts legislation and other plans. Health care is assumed to be a right for every U.S. citizen regardless of sex, creed, ability to pay, health status, and national origin. In addition to the provision of basic health care, benefits such as health promotion and long-term and rehabilitative care are provided to all participants from cradle to grave. Lifelong financial contributions to the system insure that everyone receives health care coverage.

The key to the working of the system lies in the well-organized arrangement of primary, secondary, and tertiary facilities. Existing facilities make up the new health system, but these facilities are organized in a fashion that allows the patient to enter and exit the appropriate level of care more easily. The organized system guarantees that follow-up will be effective and efficient.

The complexities associated with cancer care and financing, beginning with cancer prevention, early diagnosis, and prompt treatment, depend on a system that promotes the maximum in health care for both the provider and consumer. As we consider the burden of cancer care and costs to our nation, it is relevant to ask: "What reasonable impact on cancer could we expect with a universal, nationwide plan?"

CANCER CARE

The American health care system stands above all other nations in its potential to deliver cancer care. Yet several industrialized countries have a lower per capita cancer mortality rate (Silverberg and Lubera 1988) (see Table 16.2).

The present U.S. health care system holds a vast but unorganized, fragmented, and unnecessarily costly array of health and cancer care services. Preventive, diagnostic, treatment, rehabilitative, and reconstructive modalities are abundant, as are support and financial services. However, these services are offered by so many providers—public, private, profit, nonprofit, primary, secondary, and tertiary—that they present organizational barriers for health care professionals who attempt to deliver coordinated services, and for health care consumers who attempt to gain access to services.

Table 16.2: Cancer Around the World, 1982–83: Age-Adjusted
Death Rates per 100,000 Males Compared with 100,000 Females
for Selected Sites

Country	Males	Females
Australia	218.2	131.0
Barbados	155.7	118.4
Bulgaria	166.2	102.4
Dominican Republic	67.3	65.0
Finland	227.5	124.2
France	262.9	121.3
Germany, D.R.	214.7	132.1
Greece	160.7	100.9
Iceland	195.7	149.4
Japan	194.3	105.6
Mexico	91.5	92.8
Norway	198.3	131.6
Panama	115.1	93.5
Peru	75.8	76.3
Puerto Rico	140.3	89.6
Romania	153.6	99.7
Sweden	177.0	131.7
Switzerland	241.4	135.5
U.S.	216.6	136.5
Yugoslavia	186.1	107.8

The movement to decrease cancer through health education illustrates why our nation needs a unified health plan. Studies have shown that individuals chart their cancer course by their life-styles. In one study, some 80 percent of the lung cancer victims smoked at some time during their lives (Painter 1988). Another life-style factor—a high-fat diet—is being blamed for colon and breast cancers (U.S. Surgeon General 1979). It is important that our nation's people learn about life-styles that contribute to cancer prevention.

However, cancer education often occurs serendipitously. It amounts to being in the right place at the right time with the right attitude and the right incentive. Even though nearly 85 percent (3,020) of the 3,578 U.S. hospitals responding to a recent American Hospital Association's Center for Health Policy poll said they sponsored health promotion programs, the American public at large remains nearly untouched in this area (American Hospital Association 1985). Only 2.3 percent of American's health care dollars are spent for health promotion (Himmelstein and Woolhandler

1984). A moderately effective promotion program could save more than 6 percent of total health spending each year (Terris 1980). The Canadian National Health System, implemented in the late 1940s, demonstrates the potential for an effective nationalized health promotion plan. Boasting lower cancer mortality rates than the United States, it has spread and continues to spread the healthy life-style message. A recent nationwide effort, "Achieving Health for All: A Framework for Health Promotion," details how the unified system can better achieve equity, while promoting the health of Canadians (Epp 1986).

Not only will a national plan influence the coordinated delivery and financing of health care, but it will also affect the accessibility of comprehensive coverage. The experience of other nations with such a plan reveals that, for the most part, the universal intent stands the test. Nearly all West Germans, except for the 7 percent opting out of the system, are covered under the national system. Other countries with a nationalized system report similar results: Canada has only 5 percent of the population insured outside the national system; and England has 5 percent insured through a parallel private insurance and delivery system. In contrast, at any given time, the United States has a minimum of 16 percent and as much as 31 percent of its population living without health care coverage (Reinhardt 1987).

The ability to learn about cancer prevention, or to initiate the proper course of treatment once cancer has been diagnosed, largely determines the nature of an individual's cancer experience. Treatment to remove, radiate, or mediate cancer must be initiated in a timely fashion to fight, halt, or remove the cancer. If either cost or the inability to navigate through the system in any way delays prompt diagnosis or treatment, the greater cost for more extensive cancer care will ultimately increase the overall cancer expenditures.

With our current system, it is unlikely that we will ever reach all of the Americans who need cancer care. A universal health plan could result in a unified cancer prevention, diagnostic, and treatment campaign for the nation. As a result, cancer's deadly impact could be thwarted.

CANCER COSTS

The staggering costs for cancer care, $65.2 billion in 1985, heartily contribute to our nation's soaring health care expenditures (see

Chapter 3 by Rice, Hodgson, and Capell). Since the passage of Medicare and Medicaid legislation in 1965, numerous attempts to curb rising health care costs have met with minimal success.

A national health plan would undoubtedly curb costs for health and cancer care. A review of the U.S. and Canadian health expenditures shows that, 20 years ago, 6 percent of the gross national products of both countries went to health care. Since that time, Canadians have implemented a universal, nationwide health service system. Today, health care represents 8 percent of the Canadian GNP, but the United States, even with all of its cost-cutting measures (including DRGs), cannot boast that success. The Canadian delivery structure resembles that of the United States, but its administrative and financing systems reflect a nationalized, yet provincially run, health care system. Since none of the other 70 industrialized countries with a national health system so closely reflect the American philosophy, Canada's plan warrants further study (Roemer 1986).

HOW FAR BEYOND DRGs

Our nation's political and economic environments will be most important in charting the course of action toward a national health plan. However, it is also likely that a social/health reform movement will occur during the 1990s. Two factors support this notion.

First, social reform in the United States during the twentieth century has seemed to go in cycles of 25 to 30 years (Schlesinger 1986). Far-reaching reforms first occurred in this century between 1905 and 1912, with legislation enacting the Food and Drug Act in 1906, Worker's Accident Compensation and Mothers' Pension Benefits in 1910, and the establishment of the Children's Bureau in 1912. Some 30 years later, another cycle of major social legislative activity resulted in the Social Security Act. In 1965, the passage of the far-reaching health legislation of Medicare and Medicaid brought us into yet another cycle. If the cycle continues, we will see another far-reaching reform movement in the 1990s, possibly resulting in a national health plan.

Second, many steps toward a universal health plan have already been passed and implemented. The passage of Medicare/Medicaid in 1965 sought to provide a basic level of health care to our nation's growing elderly and poor populations. In the ensuing years, it has become evident that these programs could provide the basis for an expanded national health plan. In 1988, the passage of legislation for catastrophic health care for Medicare recipients brought us one step closer to the whole plan. Present initiatives to finance coverage of long-term care and catastrophic health care for children bring our nation even closer to the universal plan. A change in our nation's health care delivery and financing system must occur in the new decade; and it will.

CONCLUSION

Overall, our present health care system receives relatively low marks for its impact on cancer care and costs. In spite of advanced technology and warning systems, our nation's fight against cancer has not progressed as far as we desire.

A growing movement to restructure our nation's health care system could ultimately facilitate our nation's goal to reduce cancer incidence and mortality. The issue of whether a nationalized system can make a difference in cancer outcomes becomes central to support for such a system. The organization and efficiency of a skillfully planned universal, multi-entry and -exit system can foster cancer prevention activities, facilitate earlier detection of cancer, and promote more timely cancer treatment. Efforts to contain costs will bolster health promotion campaigns, enhance coordination of health services, and encourage needed levels of treatment. Today, financial and organizational barriers restrain individuals from seeking the cancer care they need. With a nationwide plan, all U.S. citizens will be entitled to receive cancer care that best ensures their happiness and productivity in the years ahead. Beyond DRGs, the fight against cancer will receive new vigor as we engage those elements of a nationwide plan that fight today's deadly killer.

REFERENCES

American Cancer Society. (1988). *Cancer Facts and Figures—1988*. New York: American Cancer Society.
American Hospital Association. (1985). "Health Promotion Programs Flourishing: Survey." *Hospitals* 59(6): 128–35.
Committee for a National Program. (1987). *Health Care Is a Right*. Rochester, NY: Coalition for a National Health System.
Dallek, G.; Hurwit, C.; and Golde, M. (1987). *Insuring the Uninsured*. Washington, DC: National Health Care Campaign.
Epp, J. (1986). *Achieving Health For All: A Framework for Health Promotion*. Ottawa, Canada: Department of National Health and Welfare.

Frieda Wolff National Health Service Fund. (1988). *RX for Our Ailing Health*. Berkeley, CA: Frieda Wolff Health Service Fund.

Gray Panthers. (1988). *It's Time for a National Health Service NOW*. Rochester, NY: Coalition for a National Health System, Special Task Force for National Health Service.

Himmelstein, D., and Woolhandler, S. (1984). "Pitfalls of Private Medicine: Health Care in the U.S.A." *The Lancet* (August 18): 391 – 94.

Massachusetts Commonwealth. (1988). House Bill 521U.

Morris, J. (1984). *Searching for a Cure*. New York: PICA Press.

National Center for Health Statistics. (1987a). "Advance Report of Final Mortality Statistics, 1985." *Monthly Vital Statistics Report* 36(5), August. DHHS Pub. No. (PHS) 86-1120. Washington, DC: U.S. Government Printing Office.

_____. (1987b). "Annual Summary of Births, Marriages, Divorces, and Deaths: United States, 1986." *Monthly Vital Statistics Report*, August. Department of Health and Human Services. Washington, DC: U.S. Government Printing Office.

_____. (1988). "Annual Summary of Births, Marriages, Divorces, and Deaths: United States, 1987." *Monthly Vital Statistics Report*, August. Department of Health and Human Services. Washington, DC: U.S. Government Printing Office.

National Health Care Campaign. (1987). *The National Health System*. Washington, DC: National Health Care Campaign.

Painter, J. (1988). "Trends and Research in Cancer." Presented at the Policy Research Project, Cancer Networks, L.B.J. School of Public Affairs, University of Texas at Austin, March.

Reinhardt, U. E. (1987). "Health Insurance for the Nation's Poor." *Health Affairs* 6(1): 101 – 12.

Roemer, M. (1986). "International Experience with National Health Insurance." Presented at the 114th Annual Meeting of the American Public Health Association, 28 September – 2 October, Las Vegas.

Schlesinger, A. (1986). *The Cycles of American History*. Boston: Houghton Mifflin.

Silverberg, E., and Lubera, J. (1988). *Cancer Statistics, 1988*. New York: American Cancer Society.

Terris, M. (1980). "Preventive Services and Medical Care: The Costs and Benefits of Basic Change." *Bulletin of the New York Academy of Medicine* 56: 180 – 88.

U.S. Surgeon General. (1979). *Report on Health Promotion & Disease Prevention*. Washington, DC: U.S. Government Printing Office.

Part VI

Cancer Care: The Ethical and Moral Issues

Newspapers and the medical literature have recently featured many articles about medical ethics. Some examine whether, in view of our limited resources, some segments of our society should be denied or given limited access to health care. Other articles discuss the issues of whether the aged should be denied sophisticated medical care and, particularly if they have a life-threatening illness, whether their treatment should consist only of measures that would allow a comfortable but early death. While our technical expertise has progressed rapidly in recent years, the appropriateness of applying these advancements to any or all members of our society has prompted discussions of the ethical considerations of such decisions. In California, during the 1988 election, the ballot contained a measure which, if passed, would have legally allowed euthanasia. It was defeated.

In Chapter 17, David C. Thomasma discusses the problem of allocation of societal resources to the patient with cancer. He observes that, as health care costs rise each year, less money is available for other societal needs. He reminds us that, by the year 2040, one-third of the population of the United States will be over 65 years of age. He also raises the issue of providing health care to the underinsured and the uninsured.

Thomasma examines these and other topics by subjecting

them to various ethical concepts. Should there be rationing of health care and, if so, by what criterion? He examines the schemes for allocation of scarce resources by applying several "theories of justice." Finally, he warns that society will suffer unless we respond to the continuing need for a national debate on these ethical considerations.

While all of the chapters in this book address cancer costs and health care considerations, Harold P. Freeman takes a unique approach in Chapter 18, focusing on the problem of delivering health care to those segments of our society that have limited or no access to such care. His subject is poverty and cancer. Freeman, the 1989 President of the American Cancer Society, draws on his experience as a provider of health care in Harlem Hospital. First, he examines cancer in various races and notes that blacks have a higher incidence and a lower survival rate than whites. He examines the statistics regarding incidence and survival in these two races for several common cancers. He then makes the point that the issue is not race but the socioeconomic status of the people involved. Poor people do not or cannot avail themselves of services for early detection or treatment of cancer and, therefore, have a lower survival rate than the affluent members of society. Poverty also leads to unemployment, inadequate education, substandard housing, chronic malnutrition, and diminished access to medical care. Finally, he lists the recommendations reported in June 1986 by the American Cancer Society's Subcommittee on Cancer in the Economically Disadvantaged. He reminds us that there are 34 million poor Americans and 37 million Americans who have no health insurance.

17 Ethical and Moral Issues in Access to Cancer Care

David C. Thomasma

ABSTRACT.   Many ethical issues in cancer care focus on clinical problems. This chapter explores another level, the macrolevel, in the ethics of cancer care. As modern technology increases, and the social will to fund high levels of cancer care diminishes, problems arise in allocation. The following schemes for allocating scarce resources are examined, along with the strengths and weaknesses of each: first come, first served; lottery; free market; social merit; volunteerism; medical triage; and social triage. Each method of allocating scarce resources is supported by one or another theory of social justice. These theories—libertarianism, egalitarianism, and maximinism—are also briefly examined. The complexity of rationing health care is enormous. Thorough discussion of all options is required in order to retain a commitment to excellence in care and compassion for those who are seriously ill.

Whenever fundamental and cherished values clash, ethical dilemmas arise. Health care in the twentieth century has had more than its share of such dilemmas. At the root of most of these dilemmas is the obligation of health professionals to act in the best interest of their patients (Beauchamp and Childress 1984). This obligation creates moral problems when other duties and rights conflict. In the field of cancer care, ethical dilemmas arise in questions about prerandomized clinical trials (Schaffner 1986), the rights of patients to refuse recommended therapy (Society for the Right to Die 1985), the use of food and water for dying patients (Lynn 1986; Thomasma, Micetich, and Steinecker 1986), requiring payment for experimental therapy, and offering unproven care for sale (Swick 1987), to name just a few.

These issues are called microissues to distinguish them from larger social issues, often called macroissues. The former arise in the clinical setting, and the latter arise in the allocation of health care. The following issues are posed in this newly expanding arena:

- The rights of all persons to expensive interventions
- The problem of the right to request experimental therapy (Thomasma and Micetich 1984)
- The question of allocation of certain scarce resources (such as Interleukin 2 in the past)
- Large-scale distribution of health care among competing health care needs (e.g., the high burdens of interventions, such as AZT, against AIDS on state public health budgets, compared to other needs such as pregnancy counseling, hypertension prevention, and the like)
- The distribution of funding to health care versus other human needs, such as defense, education, and public works

Thus, the ethics of allocating cancer care involves incredibly complex social issues. It is no surprise that the debates about access to high-technology care are played out between and among patients, health care providers, various health care services, and local, state, and federal political entities.

THE MAGNITUDE OF THE PROBLEM

Decisions about allocating access to cancer care must also take into account realities such as the cost of health care. As health care costs increase every year, less money is available for other needs in society. Yet the technological progress of modern medicine proceeds apace. Ironically, the result is that we have more to offer just when there is less money to pay for it. The taste of success has turned sour.

In addition, the gerification of society has continued. At present, there are 2.5 million people in the United States who are over 85 years old. Many of them require institutionalization. When they are hospitalized, the average cost is three times that for a person under 65 years of age. It is projected that, by the year 2040, there will be 25 million persons over 85, and one-third of the population will be over 65 (U.S. Senate 1984). Each year, then, we can expect that less money will be available to support extensive cancer care, so that increased economic and care burdens will be placed on the patients and their families in the future. What will happen 50 years from now when the number of elderly in our population will be much greater than today?

A final concern is that there is a growing number of persons in the United States who are underinsured or uninsured. It is estimated that 50 million people will suffer this problem in the near future (Durenberger 1987). When cancer strikes some of these people, as it inevitably will (one-third of all people will contract cancer at some time in their lives), access to care will be restricted by their inability to pay (Bayley 1987). The issue of justice is poignantly apparent when we consider the possibility that one person can pay for expensive therapy, such as Interleukin 2 therapy for advanced carcinoma of the intestines, while another person cannot pay for less expensive treatment. That other person may die from a Stage 2a Hodgkin's, for example, which is a potentially curable disease.

MEDICAL-INDUSTRIAL COMPLEX

The development of important drug therapies for cancer and many other diseases has led to the growth of the medical-industrial complex, as described by Arnold Relman (1981). Its effects on access to care have not yet been fully explored.

At the very least, however, the medical-industrial complex contributes to the increasingly popular view of health care as a business, which has resulted in some positive and effective management of health care costs. On the other hand, schemes that set up corporations to sell experimental or otherwise unproven therapy have had a negative impact. Quacks are not the only doctors engaged in this practice (Swick 1987).

In addition, as hospitals themselves almost adoringly adopt the business mantle, patients are correspondingly seen as consumers and physicians, providers of a product. This business model severely restricts the vision of compassion and commitment that we must have toward the sick. It contributes to the social complacency about the poor and aged who may not have proper access to care.

It also contributes to the view that institutional and professional tasks restrict rather than expand the care we owe to other human beings in our society. If we were, indeed, a poor society or one under intense stress, then we might be justified in restricting care until funding became possible. But to do so when waste, even fraud, is rampant in high levels of government is morally repugnant. The danger of the business model is that it lulls us into a false sense of accomplishment. We attain DRG targets. Our institutions survive. We are successful at cutting costs. But that success masks a terrible price in human suffering.

These considerations demonstrate the difficult problem of access to cancer care. Solutions require our best thinking. If rationing is to take place, as it is now (Reinhardt 1985), which of the various rationing schemes is the best at providing a just basis for access?

RATIONING CARE: FAIRNESS

The following are some, not all, of the schemes for allocating access to expensive cancer care therapies. Discussion of the strengths and weaknesses of these schemes assumes that access must be restricted somehow in order to contain costs. It assumes, for example, that we must address the fact that over 40 percent of the Medicare and Medicaid budget for all illnesses is spent on the last three months of persons' lives (Durenberger 1987).

First Come, First Served

One of the most effective schemes to preserve justice is to deliver care on a first-come, first-served basis. No attempt is made to judge the merit of one person's life over another, or to discriminate against a class of persons (e.g., against the aged) or against all those who have relapsed on standard therapy. Each person is treated equally, in order of arrival, until the funding runs out. Equality of treatment is also preserved until the service shuts down.

There are at least three problems with this method of allocating health care. First, some sick persons would arrive after the funding runs out. Woe to those who contract cancer near the end of the fiscal year! Second, and even more significantly, persons treated earlier (and, therefore, who have a therapeutic contract) might relapse, or need follow-up care, after funding ends. Their lives would be significantly, unacceptably endangered by delays. What is more, they might encounter some problems as the result of chemotherapeutic or radiologic interventions. It would be too much for medicine to bear the notion that the therapy's side effects could not be managed, although the initial therapy could be provided. Third, there might be an inequality of need. If one person is treated and has a stormy course (one of the 85-year-old patients who requires three times as much funding as younger patients), there might be less funding left for three persons who later contract Hodgkin's disease. Yet these three could have been cured and lived productive lives.

We may conclude that the first-come, first-served basis for allocation of care suffers from too many irremediable problems to function as a decent model of access to cancer care. It fundamentally violates the principle of medical need, which puts the needs of the patient first and allocates funds on the basis of those needs.

By Lottery

According to our present system of allocation, every time a decision is made to treat one person, someone else will be denied access. This is the dilemma now called a "tragic choice" after Calabresi and Bobbitt's celebrated analysis of the problem (Calabresi and Bobbitt 1978). Accepting this fact leads us to what seems like the only fair method of making such a choice: a lottery. Each year, people could compete by lot for the available funded slots. Perhaps this could be done by address or post office box number. During that year, persons winning the lottery would be entitled to free or discounted cancer care. All others would have to pay for their care.

The lottery also has the benefit of protecting the principle of respect for persons. No one is judged as less deserving than anyone else. Furthermore, everyone is treated fairly in the lottery, since all have an equal chance of having their number called in the draft. During each funding period, the number of slots could be adjusted according to the amount of funding available.

But the lottery idea suffers from some of the same damaging effects as the previous model. One may draw a lot but not suffer cancer that year. Perhaps one will never contract cancer but will win the lottery ten times. Others who do get cancer, and cannot afford to pay for it, would be left helplessly on the sideline.

Of course, the state might encourage altruism by soliciting donations for the needy. Americans are proud of a heritage of altruism. But recall the statistics about the gerification of society.

As people age, and do not have the same resources to pay for cancer care that they might have had when they were younger (a job and insurance), they would be less and less likely to turn in their chits to help others. This is especially prudent considering the increase in their chances of contracting some form of cancer in the future.

Thus, while appearing to be just and appearing to respect persons, the lottery is actually an allocation method that violates the principle of medical need. There would be too many "haves" who would not need the care and too many "have nots" who would need it.

Free Market

Why not continue under our current system? Why not permit access to expensive cancer care on the basis of free-market conditions? Under those conditions, competition among services and institutions would drive down costs, and persons would gain access on the basis of their ability to pay. The "safety net" could be thrown to protect those who cannot pay.

Enough has been written and said about this model. It assumes that people can pay for expensive health care. While most persons are able, through private insurance entitlement programs, to pay for their care, at least 30 to 40 million people are not able to manage this care; and it is long-term care that ruptures family budgets. Entitlement programs (such as the right to receive kidney dialysis under the Social Security law) intervene into the free market and destroy it. Furthermore, how can we believe, in the age of DRGs and government-mandated review programs, that the health care market is truly free? Economists have often pointed out that health care does not behave like other commodities. In particular, competition does not drive down costs. Costs escalate in a competitive market. Moreover, survival in a competitive market is made possible by limiting nonreimburseable patient access.

The free-market model represents a direct violation of justice. It distinguishes among persons, not on the basis of medical need, but on the basis of economics. Access is evened out only by government intervention. Even with proposals for catastrophic disease insurance, this intervention has not furthered the goal of fairness. But it is better than nothing.

Social Merit

Rather than choose those to be treated on the basis of economic merit, why not choose on the grounds of social merit? All other things being equal, that person who had best served the community would gain access to care. If tragic choices must be made, society should support the system that most encourages duties to the community. This access system carries the added benefit of permitting society to implement its goals (such as a stable family structure) through a system of positive reinforcement. To follow the example, society might give first priority for cancer care to couples who had only been married once.

This last point highlights a very real concern about social merit as an access scheme. Americans are more cautious than other people about permitting the state to determine so fully the lives of its people. In a word, social merit places an external value on the lives of citizens. Moreover, that value is set by the community, not the medical profession. The potential for abuse in a controlled society is immense, as Jay Lifton discusses in his book, *The Nazi Doctors* (Lifton 1986). Furthermore, previous experiences of allocating on the basis of social worth (the early days of kidney dialysis, for example) proved how difficult it was to decide between candidates with varying degrees of social merit: a homosexual physician, a plumber with five children, an unmarried librarian who volunteers at a community hospital, and an alcoholic poet all serve the community in their own way. It would be impossible to decide who would get cancer care, without other prejudices entering the decision.

Because the social merit method violates respect for persons by placing external values on them, violates justice by treating people unequally, and violates the real nature of a community— unity through diversity—it must be rejected as the least suitable access model. Yet we know that if a president and a bag lady came for therapy, the president would be chosen over the bag lady because of the president's presumed importance.

Volunteerism

One way to avoid all appearance of making quality of life judgments is to provide a certain minimal level of care to all persons, and then to open up any additional care only to those who volunteer for experimental therapy (Thomasma 1987). There are a number of ways to implement this scheme.

First, we could offer standard therapy for melanoma. Should that fail, volunteers for research on Interleukin 2 could obtain that therapy through federal subsidy of the research team or institute. Another way would be to aggressively treat certain forms of lung cancer by heart-lung transplant if the patient volunteers to donate a healthy heart to others. This seems to be a bizarre example, but the therapy is already used in cystic fibrosis cases. It is called "domino donation."

A third way of implementing volunteerism access might be to enlist churches and civic groups for volunteers to help with peripheral but needed aspects of care (delivering patients to radiotherapy, home visits, hospice, and the like). In return, persons would earn a place on an access waiting list in much the same way that we earn blood transfusions by donating blood. Furthermore, volunteers could be asked to sacrifice their slot for others who might need it more. Although this would be an act of pure charity, one could then begin again to earn a place on the waiting list.

Volunteerism can accomplish some of the goals of social merit without its disastrous inclusion of quality of life judgments. It encourages altruism without requiring it of everyone. As C. E. S. Wood, a Western poet and philosopher, said, "I'm from the West where . . . we believe a man has a right to go to hell if he wants to" (Oregon Historical Society 1987). Some people will not want to bother. Because a certain level of care is available to all who need it, this scheme does not violate respect for persons, justice, or the principle of medical need.

Medical Triage

At this point in the development of medical history, the principle of medical need is the only just basis for health care delivery. It involves a scheme of medical triage, whereby we treat each person according to their need. If we are forced to choose among patients due to cost cutting, we would treat those who need care the most over those who need it the least. This is how public hospitals coped with the dramatic influx of emergency room patients that occurred when the DRG system went into effect. Patients who came with heart attacks were treated, while pregnancy checkup patients (using the emergency room inappropriately as a primary care facility) were referred to neighborhood clinics.

Depending on the amount of funding, the cutoff point for treatment or referral would vary. But all persons suffering the same disease or level of disease would be treated equally. Justice as fairness would be protected, although some persons would undoubtedly suffer (those referred when nothing was available elsewhere, for example). When coupled with the volunteerism method, referrals could be made to slots voluntarily vacated by others.

One variant of medical triage would be to provide a cutoff on the basis of age (Churchill 1988). Ageism, it is pointed out, is distinguished from discrimination against sex or race by the fact that *all* persons age. A prudential system of planning for old age could include saving one's resources, knowing ahead of time that one would no longer have access to supported medical, or more specifically, cancer care. This model of "just health care," as Norman Daniels (1985) calls it, shares the good points of medical triage. It is employed in England for access to dialysis. Age cutoffs are also used in the United States (e.g., for funding heart transplants).

Ageism might be avoided in a basic medical triage model that recognizes that age should not be an independent variable in health care; rather, the variable should be medical indications. Age cutoffs are usually made on the basis of medical contraindications. Senile and debilitated persons in nursing homes who contract cancer could not withstand the rigors of an operation, radiation, or chemotherapy. Thus it seems better, from the point of view of justice, to avoid ageism in favor of medical indications.

Social Triage

Medical triage coupled with volunteerism seems to be the best model of access. However, it is hard to see how cancer care could be allocated solely on the medical triage model. Like other catastrophic diseases, it admits of little chronicity. Almost all forms of cancer will eventually result in death if they are not treated. To blacklist or "refer elsewhere" even those with skin cancer is to assign them to doom. Having cancer is not like being pregnant: we cannot send cancer patients to neighborhood clinics for care. While it may appear useless on medical grounds to place an adult leukemic who contracts pneumocysis carinii on a respirator (since such patients can rarely survive off a respirator later), medical indications alone cannot help us decide whom to treat in a class of equally seriously ill patients.

Hence, an additional model—social triage—is needed. In social triage, funding among classes of vulnerable patients is worked out ahead of time. Funding is allocated to those classes of persons who are the most in need (e.g., the catastrophically ill, the elderly poor, the retarded), before it goes to those who could, for example, alter their health profiles through life-style changes. One form of social triage is "the preferential option for the poor," in which the most vulnerable population—the poor—would receive first access to health care (O'Connell 1988).

Social triage fulfills respect for persons because quality of life judgments are not made. It fulfills the requirements of justice because all classes of citizens are treated equally. It enhances social altruism by employing volunteerism. And it contributes to a compassionate society by righting the imbalances caused by discrimination on the basis of poverty, race, age, and disease itself.

THEORIES OF JUSTICE

The line of argument so far entails a theory of justice by which different models of access are judged more or less meritorious. A great deal of dispute occurs at this level, since each access scheme is supported, in part, by a conflicting theory of justice. These are briefly examined before drawing a conclusion.

Libertarianism

The libertarian theory of justice holds that inequities are not unjust (Nozick 1974). They are simply unfortunate. Libertarians favor individual choices over social distribution. H. Tristram Engelhardt, Jr. (1986) argues, for example, that respect for autonomy not only contributes to a peaceable human community in a pluralistic age, but that such respect is a precondition for ethics. It follows that libertarians generally oppose any access scheme that deprives individuals of their rights in favor of helping others. The lottery is a favored scheme since it does not impose choices but rather leaves these to chance. Libertarians often oppose entitlement programs and taxing the rich to care for the poor. The natural lottery, however, deals some persons a more rotten hand than others. It demands a more compassionate theory of justice than libertarians can muster. Additionally, libertarianism rarely respects the concerns of health care providers for beneficent action toward patients (Pellegrino and Thomasma 1988).

Egalitarianism

A second theory holds that justice is equity (Veatch 1981). That means that each person must be treated equally. While supporting the notion of equal access to care, egalitarians do not accept any diminution of the rights of some persons for the benefit of others. Thus, they might support a scheme that gave equal access to all persons up to a maximum dollar limit, but none that distinguished among any persons on the basis of need. While certainly an improvement over the libertarian theory, from the point of view of health care objectives, this theory fails to respect the social vulnerability caused by poverty, disease, and age.

Maximinism

The third major theory is the maximin theory (Rawls 1971), which suggests that we should maximize the position of those least able (the minimum) to care for themselves. One way of doing this is to define justice as fairness. The imbalance that is "righted" is, as it were, the starting gate. We are not obligated to treat all people as if they were equal. They are not. Rather, we ensure that all receive the same opportunity to compete for the available health care goods and services (Daniels 1985).

Another version holds that justice involves more than an exchange of goods and services and the contracts that govern them. It must also concern itself with a constant and enduring attention to imbalances of power, even those that occur between the sick and their caregivers. Hence, more is required than mere equality of opportunity. Equality in relationships must also receive attention, particularly when persons who are sick have needs that transcend their ability to meet those needs (such as a cancer patient), and others (oncologists) have the power to meet those needs (Ozar 1981).

The purest form of the maximin theory is one that claims that access must first be given to the most vulnerable and neglected in an effort to right both the health care imbalance and the social imbalance implied by social class or other circumstance. This may be seen as an altruistic and optional view that sees justice as a voice of love, a work of special sacrifice for health care workers and systems.

CONCLUSION

A continued national debate on these issues could result in a national commitment toward cancer care along the lines of the combined volunteer, medical triage, and social triage models discussed in this chapter. If nothing like these models is forthcoming, then our ideals—of health care as a social good, health care institutions as social agencies, and health care workers as healers of the sick—are at even greater risk. If the most vulnerable among us do not receive special care by virtue of justice, then our society will be condemned to live by an ethic of "all persons for themselves." We will regress to a semi-civilized state, a society doomed to its own narcissism.

REFERENCES

Bayley, C. (1987). "Access to Health Care: A Case of National Schizophrenia." In *Health Care for the Uninsured: Politics, Economics, and Social Justice*, 12 – 25. Omaha, NE: Creighton University Center for Health Policy and Ethics.

Beauchamp, T., and Childress, J. (1984). *Principles of Biomedical Ethics*. 2nd ed. New York: Oxford University Press.

Calabresi, G., and Bobbitt, T. (1978). *Tragic Choices*. New York: Norton.

Churchill, L. (1988). "Should We Ration Health Care by Age?" *Journal of American Geriatric Society* 36(July): 644 – 47.

Daniels, N. (1985). *Just Health Care*. Cambridge, MA: Cambridge University Press.

Durenberger, D. (1987). "Health Care: Policy and Politics in the 100th Congress." In *Health Care for the Uninsured: Politics, Economics, and Social Justice*, 3 – 10. Omaha, NE: Creighton University Center for Health Policy and Ethics.

Engelhardt, H. T., Jr. (1986). *The Foundations of Bioethics*. New York: Oxford University Press.

Lifton, R. (1986). *The Nazi Doctors*. New York: Basic Books.

Lynn, J., ed. (1986). *By No Extraordinary Means: The Choice to Forgo Life-Sustaining Food and Water*. Bloomington: Indiana University Press.

Nozick, R. (1974). *Anarchy, State, and Utopia*. New York: Basic Books.

O'Connell, L. (1988). "The Preferential Option for the Poor and Health Care in the United States." In *Medical Ethics: A Guide for Health Care Professionals*, edited by J. Monagle and D. Thomasma, 306 – 13. Rockville, MD: Aspen Publishing Co.

Oregon Historical Society. (1987). Quotation on billboard. Portland, Oregon.

Ozar, D. (1981). "Justice and a Universal Right to Basic Health Care." *Social Science and Medicine* 15(March): 135 – 41.

Pellegrino, E. D., and Thomasma, D. (1988). *For the Patient's Good: The Restoration of Beneficence in Health Care*. New York: Oxford University Press.

Rawls, J. (1971). *A Theory of Justice*. Cambridge: Harvard University Press.

Reinhardt, U. E. (1985). "Health Care for America's Poor." *Princeton Alumni Weekly*, 27 February, 23 – 29.

Relman, A. (1981). "The New Medical-Industrial Complex." *New England Journal of Medicine* 304(4): 231 – 33.

Schaffner, K., ed. (1986). "Ethical Issues in the Use of Clinical Controls." *Journal of Medicine and Philosophy* 2(November): 297 – 316.

Society for the Right to Die. (1985). *The Physician and the Hopelessly Ill Patient: Legal, Medical and Ethical Guidelines.* New York: Society for the Right to Die.

Swick, T. (1987). "Experimental Cancer Clinic Grows and With It, the Controversy." *ACP Observer* 7(January): 1, 8 – 9.

Thomasma, D. (1987). "Ethical and Legal Issues in the Care of the Elderly Cancer Patient." *Clinics in Geriatric Medicine* 3(August): 541 – 47.

Thomasma, D., and Micetich, K. (1984). "The Ethics of Patient Requests for Experimental Therapy." *CA: A Journal for Clinicians* 34(March/April): 3 – 5. Reprinted as a monograph by the American Cancer Society, October 1984.

Thomasma, D.; Micetich, K.; and Steinecker, P. (1986). "Continuance of Nutritional Care in the Terminally Ill Patient." *Critical Care Clinics* 2(January): 61 – 71.

U.S. Senate. (1984). Special Committee on Aging, in conjunction with the American Association of Retired Persons. *Aging America: Trends and Projections.* Washington, DC: U.S. Government Printing Office.

Veatch, R. M. (1981). *A Theory of Medical Ethics.* New York: Basic Books.

18 Poverty and Cancer Care

Harold P. Freeman

ABSTRACT.   There is a significant disparity in cancer incidence and survival between black and white Americans. This chapter
discusses whether racial differences are the cause of this disparity. It
concludes that the disparity is due primarily to differences in economic
status. Reducing this disparity will require the energetic application of
culturally targeted public education to the disadvantaged, and strong
advocacy for legislative change locally and nationally, so that all Americans will be provided with adequate information and appropriate access
to screening, diagnosis, and treatment of cancer.

Any meaningful consideration of the cost of cancer
care must focus on the plight of those individuals in our society
who suffer a disproportionate cancer burden because of insufficient financial resources. It is therefore appropriate that we
explore the effect of cancer on those persons or groups who are
economically disadvantaged.

It is important to see things in their true perspective. *What
you see depends on where you stand* is a principle embodied in
the Theory of Relativity of the great theoretical physicist Albert
Einstein. Although Einstein was making reference to the observation of physical phenomena, his principle may also be applied to
sociological events. It is sometimes beneficial to look at an issue
from the outside—to stand back from where you live and work in
order to derive a clearer and more objective perception of a subject. As an illustration, note that Gunnar Myrdal, the Swedish
economist, came to this country in the 1940s and studied the
American socioeconomic system. From his point of view as an

outsider, with very few assistants and no computers, he made some assessments that proved to be accurate and of profound implication (Myrdal 1944). He predicted that significant social conflict would occur in America, a nation founded on democratic principles outlined in a constitution written more than 200 years ago. According to that document, all people are created equal. In practice, this was a sham. At the time of Myrdal's analysis there were a significant number of Americans, the former slaves, who were neither regarded nor treated as being equal. Myrdal recognized this incongruity and predicted it would result in serious social upheaval. It did!

In the 1960s, Martin Luther King, Jr. and others protested the double standard for white and black Americans and set into motion changes that resulted in the elimination of legalized segregation in America. Since then, much progress has been made, but the process is not complete. The effect of this nation's long history of perpetuation of legalized segregation is a key factor in explaining many of the health disparities that still persist between the races.

In 1973, an important study was published by Henschke et al. (1973) at Howard University Medical School. For the first time, from a national perspective, a significant disparity was established in cancer incidence and survival in black compared to white Americans. Since that time, we have focused on those differences and, more recently, have tried to determine whether or not race itself is the fundamental cause of this disparity. For a long time, many people assumed that it is. In the following discussion an attempt is made to answer this important question.

CANCER INCIDENCE ACCORDING TO RACE

Black Americans have a higher overall incidence of cancer than whites. Native Hawaiians have a very high incidence of cancer. The incidence of cancer in the native American is low (possibly because native Americans live such a short time that they do not survive long enough to develop many cancers) (Figure 18.1). With respect to selected sites, the following points are noteworthy:

- Black males have the highest incidence of prostatic cancer in the world (Figure 18.2).

Figure 18.1: Age-Adjusted Cancer Incidence Rates per 100,000
by Racial/Ethnic Group, 1978 – 81: All Sites Combined

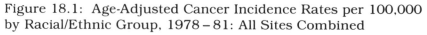

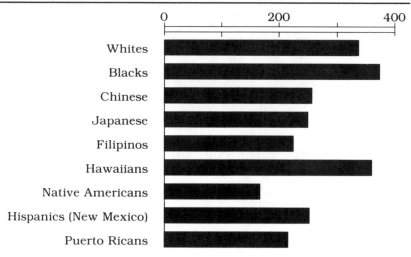

Source: U.S. Department of Health and Human Services, National Institutes of
Health, National Cancer Institute, *Cancer Among Blacks and Other Minorities*, NIH
Pub. No. 86-2785 (Washington, DC: U.S. Government Printing Office, 1986), 68.

- Breast cancer incidence is higher in white females than
  black females. Also, this cancer has a very high incidence
  in Hawaiians (Figure 18.3).
- Cervical cancer has a high rate of occurrence in blacks and
  in native Americans (Figure 18.4).
- Blacks have a higher incidence of lung cancer than whites.
  This is related to the fact that black males smoke more than
  any other sex/race group in this country. It is well known
  that smoking causes greater than 85 percent of lung cancer
  (Figure 18.5).
- Black Americans have a relatively high incidence of stomach cancer and a much higher incidence of esophageal cancer compared to whites (Figures 18.6 and 18.7).

It is noteworthy that blacks have a higher incidence of several of
the cancers that are highly lethal (lung, esophagus, and stomach),
a factor that increases relative mortality in blacks.

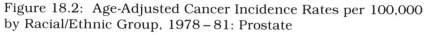

Figure 18.2: Age-Adjusted Cancer Incidence Rates per 100,000
by Racial/Ethnic Group, 1978–81: Prostate

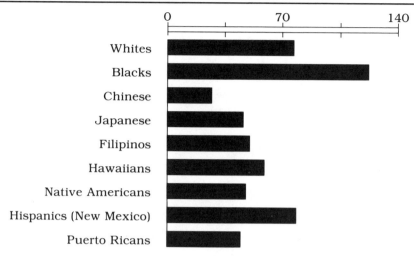

Source: U.S. Department of Health and Human Services, National Institutes of
Health, National Cancer Institute, *Cancer Among Blacks and Other Minorities*, NIH
Pub. No. 86-2785 (Washington, DC: U.S. Government Printing Office, 1986), 81.

CANCER SURVIVAL ACCORDING TO RACE

The white female has the lowest cancer mortality rate and the
highest survival rate. The black male has the highest cancer mortality rate and the lowest survival rate. In between is the white
male, who has a higher mortality rate than the black female.
Based on these statistics, one might wonder if there is a genetic
explanation for the higher death rate from cancer in blacks.

Overall, five-year cancer survival in black Americans is 38
percent, compared to 50 percent in white Americans (a significant
12 percent difference). We have pointed out the fact that native
Americans have a low incidence of cancer, but it is significant that
this population has the lowest cancer survival rate of all groups
(U.S. Department of Health and Human Services 1986). It is striking that the Japanese have a better survival rate than any racial
group in America, including whites (Figure 18.8). This finding
raises the question of whether the "minority" classifications need
special assistance. It is also interesting that Japanese Americans

Figure 18.3: Age-Adjusted Cancer Incidence Rates per 100,000
by Racial/Ethnic Group, 1978 – 81: Breast (female)

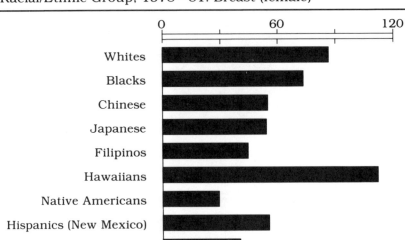

Source: U.S. Department of Health and Human Services, National Institutes of
Health, National Cancer Institute, *Cancer Among Blacks and Other Minorities*, NIH
Pub. No. 86-2785 (Washington, DC: U.S. Government Printing Office, 1986), 70.

have the highest educational indices among American racial
groups.

With respect to specific selected sites, the following points
apply:

- Survival is 75 percent for cancer of the breast in white
  Americans compared to 63 percent in blacks (Figure 18.9).

- Survival for colon cancer has a similar pattern: 52 percent
  in whites and 46 percent for blacks (Figure 18.10).

- Whites have a 68 percent five-year survival rate in cancer of
  the cervix, compared to a 63 percent survival rate in blacks
  (Figure 18.11).This disparity was previously greater and
  has been gradually reduced by the widespread increase in
  use of the Pap smear.

Survival is uniformly poor for cancer of the lung, regardless of
race. Five-year survival is 12 percent for whites and 11 percent for
blacks, reflecting essentially no racial difference (Figure 18.12).
This lack of disparity is in keeping with the reality that no effective

Figure 18.4: Age-Adjusted Cancer Incidence Rates per 100,000 by Racial/Ethnic Group, 1978 – 81: Cervix Uteri

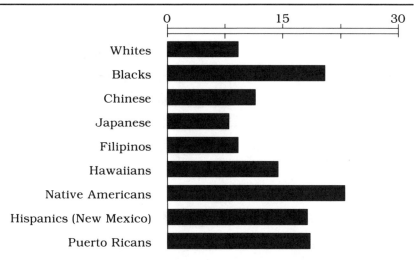

Source: U.S. Department of Health and Human Services, National Institutes of Health, National Cancer Institute, *Cancer Among Blacks and Other Minorities*, NIH Pub. No. 86-2785 (Washington, DC: U.S. Government Printing Office, 1986), 71.

method has been developed to cure lung cancer. Prevention of lung cancer is currently the only reasonable approach. It is well known that more than 85 percent of lung cancers result from cigarette smoking, an addiction that is estimated to cause about one-third of all cancer deaths in America.

For esophageal cancer, the survival rates are even worse. Blacks have a 5 percent five-year survival rate and whites, 7 percent (Figure 18.13). Medicine has not yet developed an effective treatment for this cancer either. This means that a person who develops esophageal cancer will almost certainly die from it. It is a disease that is believed to be caused by a combination of poor nutrition, cigarette smoking, and heavy intake of alcohol. Prevention of this disease requires life-style modification.

A study of 165 patients admitted to Harlem Hospital with breast cancer in the 1970s found an overall five-year survival rate of 30 percent, compared to about 60 percent for the rest of the country. The patients were all poor black Americans. In 50 per-

Figure 18.5: Age-Adjusted Cancer Incidence Rates per 100,000
by Racial/Ethnic Group, 1978 – 81: Lung

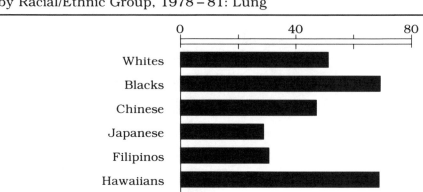

Source: U.S. Department of Health and Human Services, National Institutes of
Health, National Cancer Institute, *Cancer Among Blacks and Other Minorities*, NIH
Pub. No. 86-2785 (Washington, DC: U.S. Government Printing Office, 1986), 77.

cent of the patients, the mean delay from the first symptom of the
cancer to treatment was about one year (Freeman 1979).

CANCER IN THE ECONOMICALLY DISADVANTAGED

While it is important to collect data according to race, the question
arises as to whether population studies *based* on race offer the
best way to understand, evaluate, and influence incidence, mortality, and survival disparities. We might ask, for example, how the
combination of poverty and ignorance affects cancer incidence
and survival. With this question in mind, the American Cancer
Society assembled a Committee on Cancer in the Economically
Disadvantaged, which was charged with examining in depth the
influences of socioeconomic status (SES) on (1) risk of developing
cancer, (2) promptness in obtaining diagnosis, (3) access to and
adequacy of medical care and other factors that may contribute to
cancer incidence, mortality, and lower survival rates. The commit-

Figure 18.6: Age-Adjusted Cancer Incidence Rates per 100,000 by Racial/Ethnic Group, 1978 – 81: Stomach

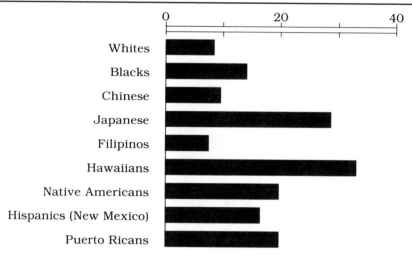

Source: U.S. Department of Health and Human Services, National Institutes of Health, National Cancer Institute, *Cancer Among Blacks and Other Minorities*, NIH Pub. No. 86-2785 (Washington, DC: U.S. Government Printing Office, 1986), 83.

tee issued its final report in 1986 (American Cancer Society 1986). Utilizing Bureau of Census figures, the special report profiles the nation's disadvantaged populations. It points out that, in a general population of 238 million, nearly 34 million (or 15 percent) live below the poverty level, which is currently about $11,200 for a family of four. This level is based on the Poverty Index created by the Social Security Administration and revised by the Federal Interagency Committee in 1980.

Those living below the poverty level include 23 million white Americans, 9.5 million black Americans, and 1.2 million other than blacks or whites. More than 12.7 million of the nation's poor live in the South; 8.3 million in the Midwest; 6.5 million in the Northeast, and 6.0 million in the West. This includes a million migrant agricultural workers (U.S. Department of Commerce 1985).

Two-thirds of the poor in America are white and about one-third are black. Thus one-third of the nation's poor are found within 12 percent of its population. Moreover, one-third of black

Figure 18.7: Age-Adjusted Cancer Incidence Rates per 100,000
by Racial/Ethnic Group, 1978 – 81: Esophagus

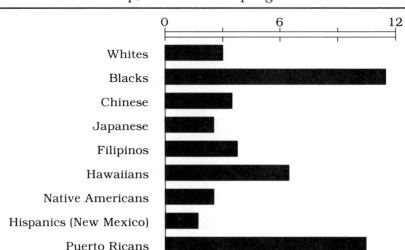

Source: U.S. Department of Health and Human Services, National Institutes of
Health, National Cancer Institute, *Cancer Among Blacks and Other Minorities*, NIH
Pub. No. 86-2785 (Washington, DC: U.S. Government Printing Office, 1986), 75.

Americans are poor. These findings underscore the disproportionate concentration of the nation's poverty in blacks, a reality that
has deep social significance.

Overlapping the nation's 34 million poor are 37 million Americans who have no health insurance. When these two groups are
combined, we observe that about 55 million Americans have difficulty in obtaining quality health care services. About 20 million of
the uninsured live above the poverty level and are comprised
mostly of working people. Another 17 million of the uninsured live
below the poverty line, meaning that one-half of the nation's poor
are not poor enough to receive medical assistance (too rich for
Medicaid but too poor for Blue Shield).

The circle of poverty is not a closed one. Some are trapped in
it for a lifetime; others escape from it; some middle-class people are
reduced to it. Cancer itself may cause impoverishment, as countless Americans are rendered poor in the course of paying for essential treatment over prolonged illnesses. These are important
observations to make in a society in which the poor are often

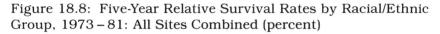

Figure 18.8: Five-Year Relative Survival Rates by Racial/Ethnic
Group, 1973 – 81: All Sites Combined (percent)

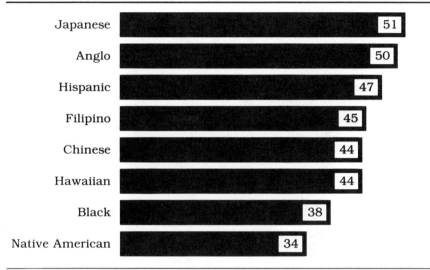

Source: U.S. Department of Health and Human Services, National Institutes of
Health, National Cancer Institute, *Cancer Among Blacks and Other Minorities,* NIH
Pub. No. 86-2785 (Washington, DC: U.S. Government Printing Office, 1986), 130.

thought of as "others" when, in reality, circumstances may
reduce anyone to poverty. We should all see ourselves reflected in
the poor.

A basic profile of the nation's poor has emerged, based on
Bureau of Census findings and other sources. The main features of
poverty that influence the problem of early detection, treatment,
and survival of cancer include: unemployment, inadequate education, substandard housing, chronic malnutrition, and diminished
access to medical care. Furthermore, poor people tend to develop a
fatalistic attitude, born of powerlessness, and to place priority on
day-to-day survival.

Consider the following illustration: A woman concerned
about food, clothing, and shelter is less likely to be concerned
about a painless lump in her breast. If the woman wanted to have
the lump examined, she would probably go to an emergency room
since she has no doctor. There she might be told, in effect, "We
have some really sick people here who are bleeding and hurting."

Figure 18.9: Five-Year Relative Survival Rates by Racial/Ethnic Group, 1973 – 81: Breast (female) (percent)

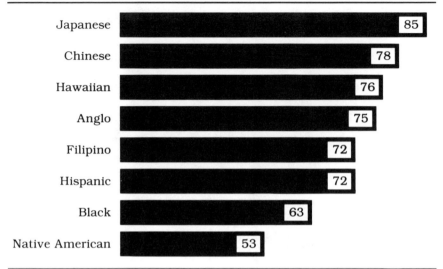

Source: U.S. Department of Health and Human Services, National Institutes of Health, National Cancer Institute, *Cancer Among Blacks and Other Minorities*, NIH Pub. No. 86-2785 (Washington, DC: U.S. Government Printing Office, 1986), 132.

So she would be referred to a clinic where she is asked to register and give proof of medical insurance, which she might not have. She might decide that the process of registration is more painful than the painless lump. In this manner, people are often triaged back to their communities, returning months later with incurable cancer. This kind of story is enacted again and again.

The committee's report concluded that the recurring cycle of poverty constitutes a key component in the problem of cancer control.

RACE IN RELATION TO CANCER

Let us look at race in relation to cancer. To date there is no genetic explanation for racial differences in cancer incidence and outcome. To the contrary, differences in cancer incidence and survival between whites and blacks appear to be largely attributable to environmental factors, including socioeconomic status.

Figure 18.10: Five-Year Relative Survival Rates by Racial/Ethnic Group, 1973 – 81: Colon and Rectum (percent)

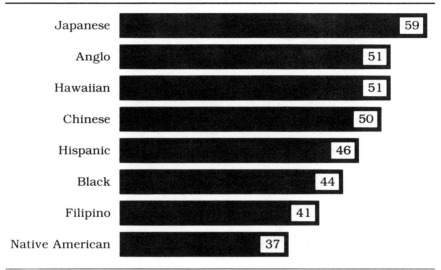

Source: U.S. Department of Health and Human Services, National Institutes of Health, National Cancer Institute, *Cancer Among Blacks and Other Minorities*, NIH Pub. No. 86-2785 (Washington, DC: U.S. Government Printing Office, 1986), 135.

Race may be seen as a gross variable for some important elements of life. For example, it may be a basis for one's cultural traditions, life-style, and belief system; and these factors do affect people's health care prerogatives and approach. Poverty is also a proxy for other elements of life, such as lack of education, unemployment, poor nutrition, substandard housing, and day-to-day survival. While neither race nor poverty is an absolute indicator of health status, each is a surrogate of predictable conditions and circumstances that may result in certain health patterns.

POVERTY, RACE, AND CANCER

Poverty is associated with a number of negative effects, including inadequate information and knowledge; inadequate physical and social environment; risk-promoting attitude, life-style, and behavior; and diminished access to health care. All of these factors contribute to decreased survival. Diminished access to health care results in low-quality and inadequate continuity of care, as well as

Figure 18.11: Five-Year Relative Survival Rates by Racial/Ethnic Group, 1973 – 81: Cervix Uteri (percent)

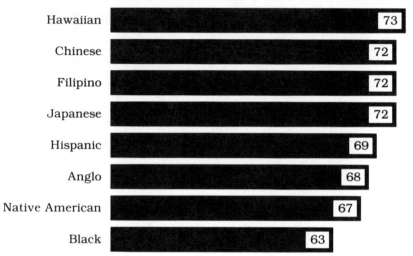

Source: U.S. Department of Health and Human Services, National Institutes of Health, National Cancer Institute, *Cancer Among Blacks and Other Minorities*, NIH Pub. No. 86-2785 (Washington, DC: U.S. Government Printing Office, 1986), 133.

insufficient access to detection, diagnosis, treatment, and rehabilitation.

How do race and poverty affect health? Poverty acts through the prism of race (culture, life-style), and the effect of poverty on the factors listed above may be modified by culture. For example, if people of a certain culture do not smoke, do not drink alcoholic beverages, and are vegetarian (as is the case with the Seventh Day Adventists), they will be protected, for the most part, from certain cancers, whether or not they are poor.

Race as a marker for culture is important, but evidence indicates that economic status prevails as a more significant surrogate of human circumstances. There are certain measurable socioeconomic indices that may provide key explanations for the disparities in cancer results (U.S. Department of Health and Human Services 1983):

Figure 18.12: Five-Year Relative Survival Rates by Racial/Ethnic Group, 1973 – 81: Lung and Bronchus (percent)

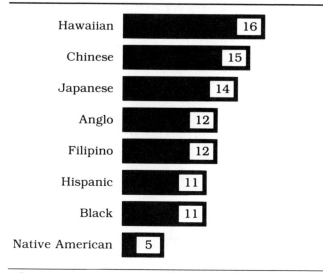

Source: U.S. Department of Health and Human Services, National Institutes of Health, National Cancer Institute, *Cancer Among Blacks and Other Minorities*, NIH Pub. No. 86-2785 (Washington, DC: U.S. Government Printing Office, 1986), 139.

Figure 18.13: Five-Year Relative Survival Rates by Racial/Ethnic Group, 1973 – 81: Esophagus (percent)

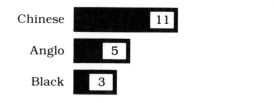

Source: U.S. Department of Health and Human Services, National Institutes of Health, National Cancer Institute, *Cancer Among Blacks and Other Minorities*, NIH Pub. No. 86-2785 (Washington, DC: U.S. Government Printing Office, 1986), 137.

1. Poverty—35 percent of black Americans are poor, compared to 12 percent of white Americans.

2. Median family income—$13,000 for black American families, $24,000 for white American families.

3. Unemployment rate—14.5 percent for blacks, 6 percent for white Americans (1986).

4. Education—78 percent of blacks and 87 percent of whites finish high school.

5. Families maintained by women alone—50 percent of black families are maintained by a woman alone versus 12 percent for white Americans (these people are among the poorest in the nation).

6. Average length of life—69 years for black Americans, 75 years for white Americans.

MAJOR FINDINGS OF THE AMERICAN CANCER SOCIETY SPECIAL REPORT

The subcommittee concluded that both cancer incidence and survival are related to SES. The subcommittee reported the following major findings:

1. In the studies that have considered SES and ethnic differences together (most based on black/white comparison), controlling for SES greatly reduces (and sometimes nearly eliminates) the apparent mortality and incidence disparities between ethnic groups. This suggests that ethnic differences in cancer are largely secondary to socioeconomic factors and associated processes.

2. There are consistent excesses of cancer mortality overall and cancer mortality for many specific sites for patients of low SES compared to high SES. It is estimated that the overall five-year survival rate of poor Americans, regardless of race, is 10 to 15 percent lower than the five-year survival of middle-class and affluent Americans.

3. Certain risk factors, behavior, dietary practices, and occupational exposures appear to be related to excess cancer incidence and mortality among economically disadvantaged persons.

4. Evidence from the American Cancer Society and other

studies has suggested that certain public myths about cancer hamper the effective use of early detection programs. Hence, targeted public education programs and the use of multimedia techniques were suggested as components in helping to eliminate this problem. At issue is the need to create educational programs that are culturally targeted to disadvantaged populations.

DISCUSSION

In 1971, the president of the United States, Richard Nixon, declared a "war against cancer." It took the form of increased resources for cancer research, primarily by a dramatic increase in funding of the National Cancer Institute. Currently, the annual budget of NCI is approximately $1.6 billion. This money is well spent since it is well known that the most profound advances await the discovery of the fundamental causes of cancer, which will ultimately lead to primary prevention. While intensifying research that may lead to cancer prevention, however, it is also necessary to apply currently known diagnostic and treatment techniques to all segments of the American population in order to achieve the highest possible cancer survival rate in light of current knowledge.

The concentration of resources on high-risk groups is an accepted medical principle in the attempt to effect substantially improved cure rates, whether in infectious disease, neoplastic disease, or other forms of illness (Freeman 1981). In a real war, military forces would be concentrated where the enemy's invasion is most aggressive and destructive. By the same logic, resources to fight cancer should be concentrated on segments of the population that are at highest risk for cancer mortality. Convincing evidence has accumulated to suggest that low socioeconomic status, regardless of race, is a major determinant of poor cancer survival. If this is so, substantial resources should be directed toward the poor and uninsured for education, diagnosis, and treatment of cancer.

The medical needs of Americans are provided by a huge economically driven medical-industrial complex, whose ultimate funding is secondary to the expenditures of a powerful, politically and economically driven military-industrial complex (with a budget of 34 percent of the gross national product). The trend in reduction of social expenditures in America is no doubt closely related to the enormous rise in military spending. The extent to which fundamental decisions concerning resources for health care are made within this perspective raises deepest concern.

Moreover, through one arm, the government is supporting the growth of tobacco and encouraging the export of tobacco to developing countries, while another government arm has shown that tobacco is overwhelmingly the most frequent cause of preventable death in America, killing 1,000 Americans every day. This is a profound conflict, which is believed to be generated by economic considerations.

A legitimate question arises as to whether or not we have properly conducted the "war against cancer." Are available resources distributed to the American people in such a way that the best survival results are obtained, or are we, as a society, aiming our guns to destroy the medical problems only of those who can pay for the guns?

It is important to stand back from where we live and work to see these issues in a proper perspective. We profess to be a society of humane people, but perhaps humanity is best measured by the manner in which we relate to the members of our society who are disadvantaged, including the poor and the elderly.

We have indicated that low socioeconomic status is a major determinant of cancer survival for the American population as a whole and is the major cause of differences in cancer outcomes between blacks and whites. The relatively poor cancer results in black Americans is an indication of the health consequences that befall a group that comprises one-tenth of the population, one-fourth of the unemployed, and one-third of the poor. But middle-class black Americans have similar results as middle-class whites. Therefore, the target population for correction of the disparity is the economically disadvantaged of any race.

In regard to cost considerations, it should be pointed out that all cancer-stricken Americans, whether rich or poor, will eventually receive care, since severely symptomatic patients are seldom denied hospital treatment. However, if treatment is ineffective because the disease is advanced, as is too often the case in the poor, the cost will be higher in dollars as well as in human suffering.

RECOMMENDATIONS

In its June 1986 report, the Subcommittee on Cancer in the Economically Disadvantaged made 49 major recommendations to the board of directors of the American Cancer Society, with a goal of reducing the disproportionate effect of cancer in the economically disadvantaged.

Listed below are selected key recommendations:

- Efforts should be made to improve the cost-effectiveness of cancer screening, with the ultimate goal of providing all at-risk Americans with this preventive measure, through advocacy and/or direct involvement.

- The cooperation of appropriate health agencies should be enlisted in a major initiative to stimulate adequate financial support and provision of health services to the economically disadvantaged.

- Adequate access should be provided to patients with signs and symptoms of cancer to promote early detection, treatment, and rehabilitation, regardless of ability to pay.

- Direct and indirect funding mechanisms should be developed to screen indigent populations at high risk for specific cancer sites.

- Emergency rooms and clinics should have outreach programs, including mobile vans for screening purposes. Persons in high-risk categories, who present themselves for treatment of other illnesses at primary care clinics and emergency rooms, should be encouraged to avail themselves of facilities for cancer screening.

- Federal and state governments should consider the feasibility of assuming responsibility for insurance programs for catastrophic illness.

- Since any improvement in the health care system must ultimately depend on the will of the American people, they must be made aware of the importance of financing early diagnosis, treatment, and rehabilitation for everyone, but especially its importance for the economically disadvantaged.

- The recording of socioeconomic status and ethnicity should be included in all epidemiological and clinical research conducted by the ACS, the NCI, and the National Center for Health Statistics.

- A study should be undertaken of factors affecting prognosis and survival for the economically disadvantaged (i.e., compliance, nutrition, home environment).

- Studies should be made to determine the most effective strategies for cessation of smoking among the economically disadvantaged.

- Additional research is needed on the factors affecting cancer incidence and survival in Hispanic, Asian, and other populations.

- Examination is needed of factors that influence the seeking of medical care to determine if there are differences according to socioeconomic status, racial, or ethnic composition.

- Funding is needed for research on the development of exploratory investigations leading to major studies of possible correlations between economically linked biochemical or immunological differences in malignant growth.

- Materials should be designed to reflect—through photos, drawing, and writing—the socioeconomic composition and ethnic diversity of our country.

- A profile of each community should be developed to facilitate program planning and implementation. The principles of the community expansion program should be integral to encouraging people in behavior modifications that might help reduce the risk of cancer.

- Materials and program delivery methods for volunteers and ACS staff should be relevant to these targeted groups.

- An emphasis should be placed on encouraging life-style and behavior changes that might help reduce the risk of developing cancer.

- A major effort should be made to educate health professionals about the important role of socioeconomic factors in the incidence and mortality of cancer (cervix, prostate, lung, esophagus, larynx, and oral sites), since many of these sites lend themselves to risk reduction through altering measures such as smoking and drinking.

- Strategies should be developed to enlist and train the economically disadvantaged to serve as volunteers in their own communities.

• Innovative communication strategies should be devised to reach the economically disadvantaged with cancer control messages.

CONCLUSION

There are 34 million poor Americans. Regardless of race, poor Americans have a 10 to 15 percent lower five-year survival rate from cancer, as well as higher cancer incidence, compared to other Americans. The racial disparities in cancer results are due primarily to differences in economic status. There are 37 million Americans who have no health insurance. These Americans have diminished access to early diagnosis and treatment of cancer. When these two overlapping segments of the population are combined, there are 55 million Americans who experience significant difficulties in seeking medical care.

Nearly 1 million Americans develop cancer and nearly 500,000 Americans die from cancer each year. A disproportionate number of people who develop cancer and die from the disease are among the economically disadvantaged of all races.

In 1983, the war against cancer took on a new approach when the National Cancer Institute set a goal to diminish the mortality from cancer by 50 percent by the year 2000. The achievement of such a goal requires, among other things, the dramatic narrowing or elimination of the gap in cancer survival between economically disadvantaged and other Americans. Substantially reducing this disparity by the year 2000 will require the energetic application of culturally targeted public education for the disadvantaged and strong advocacy for legislative change, locally and nationally, so that all Americans will be provided with adequate information and appropriate access to screening, diagnosis, and treatment of cancer.

In the words of the great civil rights leader Martin Luther King, Jr., "Of all the forms of inequality, injustice in health is the most shocking and inhumane."

REFERENCES

American Cancer Society. (1986). Cancer in the Economically Disadvantaged." Special Report prepared by the American Cancer Society Subcommittee on Cancer in the Economically Disadvantaged. New York: American Cancer Society.

Freeman, H. P. (1979). "Affirmation Action in the Diagnosis and Treatment of Cancer in Blacks." Paper presented at the American Cancer Society's Twenty-First Science Writers' Seminar, Daytona Beach, Florida.

_____. (1981). "Cancer Mortality: A Socioeconomic Phenomenon." Paper presented at the American Cancer Society's Twenty-Third Science Writers' Seminar, Daytona Beach, Florida.

Henschke, U. K.; Leffall, L. D.; Mason, C.; Reinhold, A. W.; Schneider, R. L.; and White, J. E. (1973). "Alarming Increase of Cancer Mortality in the U.S. Black Population (1950 – 1967)." *Cancer* 31(4): 763 – 68.

Myrdal, G. (1944). *An American Dilemma: The Negro Problem and Modern Democracy.* New York/London: Harper and Brothers.

U.S. Department of Commerce. (1985). *Statistical Abstract of the United States: Current Population Reports on Growth, Distribution, and Composition of American Families.* U.S. Department of Commerce. Bureau of Census. Washington, DC: U.S. Government Printing Office.

U.S. Department of Health and Human Services. (1983). *Health Characteristics according to Family and Personal Income.* Vital Health and Statistics, Series 10, No. 147. Department of Health and Human Services. Pub. No. (PHS) 85-1575. Washington, DC: U.S. Government Printing Office.

_____. (1986). *Cancer Among Blacks and Other Minorities.* Department of Health and Human Services. National Cancer Institute. NIH Pub. No. 86-2785.

Part VII

Conclusion

19 Cancer Care and Cost: Where Do We Go From Here?

Richard M. Scheffler, Kathryn A. Phillips, and Neil C. Andrews

The chapters in this book demonstrate the complexity of the problems we face in financing cancer care in the United States. The establishment of DRGs has raised a number of issues that require constant monitoring and carefully thought-out plans for the future. The contributions to this book also document the huge economic cost of cancer to society as well as the increasing threat to individual well-being.

Practitioners, policy analysts, and researchers have an enormous task in their attempt to resolve the issue of cancer care and cost. They must recognize the connection and the implicit trade-offs between the care and prevention of cancer and the resulting cost to society. These trade-offs, although they affect all areas of health policy, are undoubtedly more severe in the case of cancer. Although no agenda can anticipate every change that will occur, the material in this book suggests certain directions for future work on cancer care and cost.

The treatment of cancer patients, especially the elderly, has been dramatically affected by DRGs. Cancer discharges and lengths of stay among Medicare patients have dropped dramatically. We need to determine whether cancer treatment has been altered to the detriment of the patient. At this point, studies on the quality and outcomes of treatment have not shown whether cancer patients have been adversely affected. Long-term studies on quality of care and treatment outcomes should be given highest priority in our strategies for the future.

The cost of cancer varies systematically by site and by stage of treatment. The DRG system does not adequately consider the severity of illness and the need for treatment. There is more work to be done on the severity of cancer within DRG groups so that reimbursement policies can account more accurately for the cost of care. As cancer research develops and more technology is used in treatment and prevention, severity adjustments will be even more important. We strongly suggest that severity adjusters be developed and empirically tested for cancer DRGs.

Research should also be done on the variability of cancer costs by cancer site. We need more information on the reasons for these differences. The differences in cost between sites might be attributable to changing patterns of disease, new treatments, increased use of outpatient settings, or other reasons. By exploring these differences, we can determine whether we are truly achieving cost savings for particular sites, and if so, whether there are strategies that can be applied to achieve similar results with other sites.

Variability exists not only in costs for different sites and stages of treatment, but also in costs for different age groups, geographic areas, and people in different socioeconomic groups. In our search for efficient and equitable solutions to the high costs of cancer care, we must consider the reasons for these differences in costs and their effects on patients.

Basic research on the prevention and early treatment of cancer is, by all accounts, the most important element in any agenda to address cancer care and cost. We must be sure that DRGs and other reimbursement policies do not interfere with this work. Clinical trials should be exempt from the prospective payment system; PPS rates should encourage new treatments and preventive services; and providers should not be financially discouraged from trying to treat each patient as an individual. We suggest that committees should be formed at the national level to monitor the treatment of cancer patients. These committees would help ensure that ethical treatment of cancer patients is considered along with cost savings programs.

Finally, it is clear that the issue of cancer care and cost reflects broader changes in the U.S. health care system. Both the financing and the delivery of health care services have changed in the United States, and these changes are probably here to stay.

Therefore, we must approach our work on cancer with the knowledge that cancer care is an inextricable part of a larger system. To do this, we need researchers who are trained in interdisciplinary approaches and who are willing to work with representatives from a variety of disciplines. We need patients, providers, and third parties who are willing to work together as partners to address these issues. It is only by working together that we can seek the answers to the issue of cancer care and cost.

Index

List of Contributors

Mary S. Baker, Ph.D., is a staff scientist in the Cancer Prevention Research Program at the Fred Hutchinson Cancer Research Center, Seattle, Washington. She received her training in cancer control during an internship as a Cancer Control Science Associate at the National Cancer Institute.

Lester Breslow, M.D., M.P.H., is Dean Emeritus and Professor, School of Public Health, and Director, Health Services Research, Division of Cancer Control, Jonsson Comprehensive Cancer Center, University of California, Los Angeles (UCLA).

Frank Capell is an epidemiologist at the Office of AIDS, California Department of Health Services.

Harold P. Freeman, M.D., is Director of the Department of Surgery, Harlem Hospital Center, New York City, and Professor of Clinical Surgery, Columbia University College of Physicians and Surgeons, New York City. He served as President of the American Cancer Society in 1989. Freeman is a Diplomate of the American Board of Surgery, a Fellow of the American College of Surgeons, a senior member of the Commission on Cancer, and a Governor of the American College of Surgeons. He is on the Executive Council of the Society of Surgical Oncology, and has served as Chairman of the Surgical Section of the National Medical Association and as a consultant to the National Cancer Institute, including six years as a member of the NCI Breast Cancer Task Force. Freeman initiated a free Breast Examination Center in Central Harlem, funded by a grant from the New York State Department of Health. He has lectured extensively throughout Africa, the Middle East, and the United States on numerous subjects related to surgical oncology.

James O. Gibbs, Ph.D., is Director of Product Research and Evaluation for the Blue Cross and Blue Shield Association. He is responsible for evaluating methods of controlling the cost of health insurance benefits.

Brian S. Gould, M.D., is Senior Vice President and Medical Director of Blue Cross of California. He also serves as a Commissioner on the California Health Policy and Data Advisory Commission. Gould was educated at Johns Hopkins University and received his medical training at the University of California, San Francisco and the Pacific Presbyterian Medical Center, also in San Francisco. He is a Diplomate of the American Board of Psychiatry and Neurology and a Fellow of the American Psychiatric Association.

Thomas A. Hodgson, Ph.D., is Chief Economist in the Office of Analysis and Epidemiology at the National Center for Health Statistics, Hyattsville, Maryland. He has published numerous articles on disease-specific costs of illness and refinements in cost-of-illness methodology.

Stephen F. Jencks, M.D., M.P.H., is Senior Research Physician and Acting Director, Office of Research, Health Care Financing Administration.

Larry G. Kessler, Sc.D., is Chief of the Operations Research Section at the National Cancer Institute of the National Institutes of Health. His research, and the research of the section, includes projections of cancer incidence and mortality, modeling the effects of cancer control activities on health outcomes, issues related to cost and economics and cancer prevention and control, and national surveillance of knowledge, attitudes, and behavior with respect to cancer.

Martha Kathryn Key, Ph.D., is Director of Research and Development of EQUICOR, Inc. She is a licensed clinical-community psychologist and maintains an adjunct associate professorship in psychology at Vanderbilt University.

James Lubitz, M.P.H., is Chief of the Analytical Studies Branch of the Office of Research, Health Care Financing Administration. He is currently involved in a project to develop nationwide data on the use and outcomes of hospital care for Medicare enrollees.

Lonna T. Milburn, Ph.D., is a Lecturer and Project Director at the Lyndon B. Johnson School of Public Affairs, University of Texas at Austin. She directs projects on access to health care and cancer networks as a health delivery alternative.

Janice M. Moore, M.P.H., is a consultant in utilization and quality management and heads her own firm based in Evanston, Illinois.

She was Director of Utilization Review for the Blue Cross and Blue Shield Association for 11 years and works closely with major health care associations and third-party payers in utilization review and quality assessment.

Robert D. Narkiewicz, Ph.D., provides health care services as a private consultant. Formerly, he was Regional Director with the Admar Corporation, a health care management firm.

David J. Ottensmeyer, M.D., is Executive Vice President and Chief Medical Officer of EQUICOR, Inc. He serves as Chairman of Lovelace Medical Center, Lovelace Health Plan, and Lovelace Medical Foundation. He is past president of the American Group Practice Association and the American College of Physician Executives.

Gary A. Ratkin, M.D., is in the private practice of medical oncology and hematology and is Clinical Associate Professor of Medicine at Washington University in St. Louis, Missouri. He was Chairman of the Clinical Practice Committee of the American Society of Clinical Oncology from 1985 until 1988. He is the editor of and a contributor to *Guidelines on Successful Oncology Office Practice*.

Dorothy P. Rice, Sc.D. (Hon.), is a Professor in Residence in the Department of Social and Behavioral Sciences with joint appointments with the Institute for Health and Aging and the Institute for Health Policy Studies at the University of California, San Francisco. From 1976 until 1982, Rice was Director of the National Center for Health Statistics, where she led in the development and management of a nationwide health care information system, which is accepted and utilized by the entire health field, both public and private sectors. She is the author of more than 100 published articles and monographs on medical economics, cost of illness, aging, and health statistics.

Gerald F. Riley, M.S.P.H., is a research analyst in the Division of Beneficiary Studies, Office of Research, Health Care Financing Administration. His research interests include Medicare utilization in the last years of life and enrollment of Medicare beneficiaries in health maintenance organizations. He is currently participating in efforts to link Medicare utilization data to cancer registry data maintained by the National Cancer Institute.

Leonard D. Schaeffer is President and Chief Executive Officer of Blue Cross of California. He has served as Assistant Secretary for Management and Budget in the Department of Health, Education and Welfare (HEW), as Administrator of the Health Care Financing

Administration (HCFA) in the Department of Health and Human Services, and as President of Group Health, Inc., one of the largest health maintenance organizations in the Midwest.

Stuart O. Schweitzer, Ph.D., is Professor of Health Services, School of Public Health, University of California, Los Angeles (UCLA). His major teaching and research activities are in the areas of health care technology assessment and policy analysis.

Robert C. Smucker, M.A., is a senior programmer and statistical analyst with IMS, Inc. He works closely with National Cancer Institute investigators, providing technical and programming support for a variety of research projects.

Richard J. Steckel, M.D., is Director of the Jonsson Comprehensive Cancer Center at the University of California, Los Angeles (UCLA), and Professor of Radiological Sciences and of Radiation Oncology at the UCLA School of Medicine. He has been a consultant for a number of years to the National Cancer Program, participating in the planning of cancer centers and NCI-sponsored cancer control activities. He serves on the Board of Directors of the California Division of the American Cancer Society, and he has served as National President of the Association of American Cancer Institutes, comprising the directors and senior leadership staff of major cancer research centers in the United States.

David C. Thomasma, Ph.D., is the Fr. Michael I. English, S.J. Professor of Medical Ethics and Director of the Medical Humanities Program at Loyola University of Chicago Medical Center. He is the editor of *Theoretical Medicine* and section editor of *The Journal of the American Geriatrics Society*. He serves on the ethics advisory committees of the American Hospital Association and the Catholic Health Association.

Carol S. Viele, R.N., M.S., is Clinical Nurse Specialist in Hematology/Oncology and Bone Marrow Transplant at the medical center at the University of California at San Francisco. She is Assistant Clinical Professor in the Department of Physiological Nursing at the university and has served as a member and chairman for two years of the university's Committee on Human Research.

Charles H. White, Ph.D., is Executive Director of the medical staff of Grossmont District Hospital, a 430-bed facility in La Mesa, California. He has served as Senior Vice President of the California Hospital Association and was Program Director of the California Regional Medical Program.

About the Editors

Richard M. Scheffler, Ph.D., is a Professor of Health Economics and Public Policy at the Schools of Public Health and Public Policy, University of California, Berkeley, and is also the head of the Health Policy and Administration Program. He served as a member of the Health Financing Study Group established by the American Cancer Society, California Division.

Neil C. Andrews, M.D., is Professor Emeritus, Department of Surgery, University of California, Davis. He is immediate past president of the California Division of the American Cancer Society and continues as an active participant in that organization. Prior to joining the University of California, he was a Professor of Thoracic Surgery at Ohio State University, Columbus, Ohio. He is a member of a number of professional organizations, including the California Medical Association, and is a founding member of the American Society of Clinical Oncology and the Society of Thoracic Surgeons.

Kathryn A. Phillips, M.P.A., is a National Center for Health Services Research Predoctoral Fellow at the University of California, Berkeley. She is studying toward a Ph.D. in Health Services Research and Policy Analysis. She is also a Fellow with the American Cancer Society, California Division.